Every woman should have a friend like Dr. Hilda Hutcherson . . .

"Dr. Hilda Hutcherson delivers the kind of frank, down-to-earth information about sex and sexuality that so many of us need and crave. [She tells you] everything you always wanted to know about sex but were afraid to ask. With facts, drawings and plenty of plain-spoken advice, this is a great book to share with your daughter when it's time to have 'the talk.'"

—Linda Villarosa, author of *Body & Soul:*
The Black Woman's Guide to Physical Health and Emotional Well-Being

"Answers questions that women would like to ask their gynecologists. An honest and detailed book covering all aspects of female sexuality. An extremely valuable addition to any woman's library."

—Rogerio A. Lobo, M.D.,
Sloane Hospital for Women,
Columbia University College of Physicians & Surgeons
and New York-Presbyterian Hospital

"Her approach is so thorough and the writing so reassuring that even readers who would otherwise never pick up a sex manual will likely be comfortable with—and grateful for—this book." —*Publishers Weekly*

"The ultimate source book." —*Latina* magazine

"An honest, straightforward guide." —*Upscale* magazine

"Comprehensive yet neither confusing nor overwhelming . . . user-friendly and [an] easy read." —*Library Journal*

What Your Mother Never Told You About

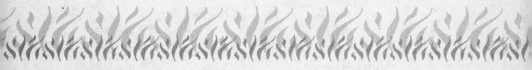

S·e·x

Hilda Hutcherson, M.D.

A PERIGEE BOOK

A Perigee Book
Published by The Berkley Publishing Group
A division of Penguin Putnam Inc.
375 Hudson Street
New York, NY 10014

G. P. Putnam's Sons hardcover edition: April 2002
First Perigee edition: February 2003

Perigee ISBN: 0-399-52853-9

Visit our website at www.penguinputnam.com

The Library of Congress has catalogued the
G. P. Putnam's Sons hardcover edition as follows:

Hutcherson, Hilda.
What your mother never told you about sex / Hilda Hutcherson.
p.   cm.
Includes bibliographical references and index.
ISBN 0-399-14842-6
1. Sex instruction for women.   2. Women—Sexual behavior.   3. Sex.   I. Title.
HQ46 .H835   2002   2001048899
613.9'6—dc21

Printed in the United States of America
10

This book is dedicated to my mother, Bernice,
who encouraged me to always follow my dreams.

Acknowledgments

A special thank you to Susan L. Taylor for planting the seed for this book; Tamara Jeffries, an exceptional writer, editor, and friend for her guidance; Miriam Biddelman, an incredible sex therapist and buddy for her expertise and caring spirit; and Judith Cummins for her realistic illustrations.

Thanks to the following writers, editors, and friends for their assistance and advice: Hilary Beard, Valerie Boyd, Ayana Byrd, Synitra Hutcherson, Alex Simmons, Holly Taylor, Linda Villarosa, and expert physical trainer Robert Corbellini.

I am grateful to the following sex-sensitive physicians who answered my many questions: Aristotelis Anastasiadis, M.D.; Gerald Hoke, M.D.; Nabil Husami, M.D.; Sylvia Karasu, M.D.; Alan Kling, M.D.; Roger Lobo, M.D.; Henry Lodge, M.D.; John Postley, M.D.; and Paula Randolph, M.D. Thanks also to the following sex and couples therapists and psychologists for their expert advice: Elana Katz, M.S.W.; Risa Ryger, Ph.D.; and Michael Perelman, Ph.D. My research was made much easier by the assistance of Amy Levine, the knowledgeable librarian at SIECUS (Sexuality Information and Education Council of the United States), Barbara Griswold, and many of my wonderful patients.

Thank you Carla Glasser—you are the world's best agent. A million thanks to my wonderful editor, Sheila Curry Oakes, who saw my vision when others didn't. Thanks Hillery Borton for your excellent editing and patience.

My greatest thanks go to my family—husband, Fredric Fabiano, and children, Lauren, Steven, Andrew, and Freddie—for their understanding and support. I love you much.

Contents

Part III: Taking Care of Yourself

Part IV: Sex for Life

Part V: When Sex Isn't Great

Preface

It was billed as the greatest day of my life by the man who was to be my husband. The room was toasty warm and filled with the sweet fragrance of roses. Soft music played. I'd planned for months for this moment. My "woman-of-the-world" roommate had taught me about birth control pills. I'd survived my very first visit to the university gynecologist. I was desperately in love and ready to give this perfect man the gift of my virginity.

He touched me slowly and gently. Softly. Lovingly. And as his hand brushed my breasts, my mother's "bad-girl" face appeared out of nowhere. "Good girls don't." . . . "Sex is only to please your husband." . . . "Don't let boys touch you." . . . "Keep your skirt down and your panties up." His hands touched my essence. Warm breath and moist kisses covered me. And as he neared my intact hymen, my preacher's "Thou-shalt-not" face materialized. "Fire and brimstone" . . . "Hell and damnation" . . . "Sin, sin, sin."

I dared not move. I dared not breathe. And just as Grandma's "Boys-are-no-good" face appeared, it was over.

"Are you all right?" He cradled me in his sweaty arms.

"I love you."

"I love you too."

I stared at the ceiling as silent tears scorched my face. Years would pass before I was confident enough to give myself permission to be a "bad girl" and celebrate the power of my sexuality.

The foundation of our sexuality and how we feel about sex is laid during childhood. Verbal and nonverbal messages from our parents, religious teachings, our culture and society all meld together to shape the sexual being that we are as adults. Traditionally it has been the job of the mother to teach daughters about sex; however, few women feel comfortable talking in detail about it. Don't blame Mom though, as it is unlikely that her mother was able to give her the complete story about sex. After all, mothers are a product of their environment. And many stories, myths, misconceptions, or complete silence have been passed down from generation to generation.

Most women assume that when it comes to the technique of lovemaking, their men will teach them all they need to know. What happens if your partner is a woman? What if your man doesn't have a clue? And who is teaching the men? Many boys learn about sex from their friends, and some depend on movies for the intimate details of making love.

In the twenty years that I have been an obstetrician and gynecologist, I have met thousands of women of every race, ethnic group, age, and socioeconomic class in America, and I have found that women's experience of sex is universal. We all share the same fears, myths, misconceptions, concerns, hang-ups, desires, needs, joys, and pleasures. Over the years, I have been asked time and time again to recommend a book that answered the basic questions that women have about sex. I studied what was available and found books that promised to teach you how to achieve hot sex, magnificent sex, mind-blowing sex, all-night sex, and incredibly outrageous sex. In my experience, most women would be happy if they got consistently satisfying, "good-enough" sex. A sprinkling of incredibly, outrageous, mind-blowing sex once in a while would be a wonderful bonus.

As women, we spend our lives thinking about and taking care of everyone else. Even when it comes to sex, many women feel that their partner's satisfaction is much more important than their own. Magazines at the checkout counters of every grocery store scream headlines expounding how to drive your man crazy in bed, how to make him beg for more, how to rope him, keep him, get him up, and get him off. Believe me, I agree that making your partner happy is important, but I also think that you need to spend just as much time and effort finding out how to increase the odds that you will be sexually satisfied as well. You must take responsibility for your own pleasure, because sexual satisfaction is your birthright.

Women are under a tremendous pressure to look perfect. When we fall short of society's look-of-the-moment, we don't feel attractive or sexy and have difficulty achieving the level of sexual pleasure that we are entitled to. Sadly many women are blind to the fact that the female body is beautiful. How did we allow "them" to convince us that women's bodies should look like that of a preadolescent boy? In an attempt to achieve a body type that is totally unnatural for most of us, we develop eating disorders, rob our bodies of nutrients, disturb our natural menstrual cycle, decrease our estrogen levels, and increase our levels of unhappiness and discontent. We worry about how we look during sex rather than how we feel. Often when I give a mirror to a woman to look at her sexual anatomy, she expresses displeasure and fails to appreciate the beauty, grace, power, and complexity of her female genitals. How did we allow "them" to convince us that our vaginas smell bad and have no feeling or that our vulvas are ugly or that the clitoris is the size of a small pea? Learning to love your self is the first step to enjoying sex and creating a fulfilling sex life. This book is written to give women the knowledge they need to begin to appreciate the wonders of female anatomy and sexuality. Chapters 1 and 2 take a look at the wondrous and exquisitely beautiful female body.

Ask a hundred women, "What is sex?", and it is likely that the majority will answer "intercourse." Yet many women receive no physical pleasure from intercourse. Expanding the definition of "sex" gives women options and the opportunity to find out what gives them the most pleasure. Chapters 4–12 present different ways that women may choose to express themselves sexually—and increase their sexual satisfaction.

In my practice, it is not unusual to see women who move between relationships with men and women during various life stages. According to the Hite Report, at least 17 percent of women have experienced sex at least once with another woman. Falling in love with a woman can be exhilarating and liberating but may sometimes be met with disapproval from family and others. Every woman, however, has the right to determine how she expresses her sexuality. In Chapters 7 and 9, I have included descriptions of specific sexual techniques that can be used when making love to a woman. And though this book is written primarily for women in opposite-sex relationships, most of the information applies equally to women-loving-women. It is impossible to cover the many dimensions of same-sex relationships and sexuality in this book, so I refer the reader to two excellent books listed in the resources section.

One of the keys to healthy sexuality is a healthy body. Chapters 13–15 discuss strategies for improving your sex life by improving your health and taking control of your body.

Female sexuality is not static; it changes over your lifetime. Pregnancy and menopause can significantly change the way a woman expresses her sexuality. Chapters 16 and 17 discuss how to keep the fires burning through these important life stages. Chapter 18 provides tools you can use to help your daughter grow up sexually healthy as well as happy and secure with her sexuality. We *can* break the cycle of myths, misconceptions, and untruths about female sexuality.

Satisfying sex can prolong your life and has been shown to decrease your blood pressure, decrease stress, strengthen your heart, and boost your immune system. Yet according to the NHSLS (National Health and Social Life Survey), 43 percent of women have sexual dysfunction. Mainstream medical journals have featured articles expounding the importance of sexual satisfaction in women's health and encouraging doctors to investigate the sexual problems of women. Pharmaceutical companies and researchers are working furiously to find a magic pill that will guarantee sexual ecstasy for every woman. While the attention to women's sexual issues is welcome, it is important that we don't make sex one more disease that needs to be treated. Chapters 19–22 discuss the many reasons that sex may not be great and offer tips to help you improve your sex life.

The keys to great sex are simple: feeling good about yourself, understanding how your body works—and that of your partner, knowledge of basic sexual techniques, willingness to experiment and ask for what you want, and, of course, caring and respect from your partner.

Part I

Body
Parts

Chapter 1

Getting to Know You

When was the last time you took a good look at your vulva? I'm not talking about anything clinical, kinky, or even sex-related—just taking a hand mirror and inspecting your genitals the same way you might examine your hands while you're doing your nails or look at your skin in the mirror when you wash your face. If you're like most women, looking at your genitals is probably not part of your usual routine. In fact, as children, most of us were taught not to look at, talk about, touch, or pay too much attention to our genitals at all. "Down there" was a private place. Additionally, female genitalia is naturally hidden—enveloped in soft folds of skin, covered by hair, and rather tucked away between our thighs—so it's no wonder our vulva has become a mystery—even to ourselves.

Beyond the woman-to-woman talk about menstruation, most mothers never sit down and describe the details of the vulva, vagina, or clitoris. (In defense of our moms, they may not know very much about the female body themselves.) Schools teach us more about dissecting frogs or turning proper French phrases than about the human body. In health class, the female sexual anatomy is not well taught: The conversation is reduced to talk of zygotes and dividing cells, accompanied by textbook graphics that rarely look like what we see between our legs. As girls, when we weren't trying to hide our developing bodies, we were whispering and giggling about sex, absorbing misinformation from friends who knew as little as we did. Magazines give ten tips for better sex, and novels describe heart-pounding accounts of sexual ecstasy, but these "resources" say little about the bodies involved—ours.

As we get older, we may listen to male sexual partners who claim to have been around. Unfortunately many men know little about their own bodies and considerably less about ours. Because many of us have been conditioned since childhood through verbal and nonverbal cues to think of our genitals as ugly, smelly, and unclean, we aren't able to fully enjoy intimate encounters because of fear that our partner will be turned off by the sight, smell, and taste of our genitals. Unlike men, who experience a veritable show-and-tell in the locker room, we can't compare our genitals to other women's. Unfortunately, we are often left wondering if our genitals are "normal."

We have few means of discovering the tremendous variability of the female sexual anatomy and discovering the truth about the fabulous female body. After years of ignoring that mysterious area "down there," it's no wonder we come to think of our genitalia as inferior, unattractive, unmentionable, and abnormal. When I pick up a hand mirror and ask the women who come to my office to look at their sexual anatomy, a too-common response is "Yuck! It's ugly" or "Am I normal?" I have never heard a woman exclaim "How beautiful!" Yet the female anatomy is exquisitely designed, miraculous, and beautiful. Getting to know your sexual body is vital for your physical health and sexual well-being because the more you know about your body, the more ways you'll discover to obtain pleasure and greater sexual gratification—and the more likely you are to know when something is amiss with your sexual health or sexual functioning. I find that when women begin to learn about their bodies and they begin to feel more comfortable with how their vagina acts and responds, they're intrigued by it—and usually quite empowered to take more control of their well-being—sexual and otherwise.

The Vulva

The part of your sexual anatomy that you can see is called the *vulva*—the external part of the genitals that includes the *mons, labia minora, labia majora,* and the *clitoris.*

To begin your examination of your vulva, find a well-lit room and grab a mirror. Sit at the edge of a chair or prop yourself up on pillows on a bed, then arrange the light and the mirror so that your hands are free and you have a clear view of your vulva. If you've never taken a look at your genitals before, don't be surprised if you don't find them particularly attractive; your vulva is moist and hairy with textures, colors, and aromas unlike those found on any other part of your body. Learning to admire and appreciate your sexual anatomy will make it easy for you to accept, enjoy, and experience the full potential of your sexuality.

The Mons

The *mons pubis,* or *mons,* is a cushion of fat on top of the pubic bone that is covered with skin and hair. The hair begins to grow in as you hit puberty—around eleven or twelve years old. (We are not sure why we have

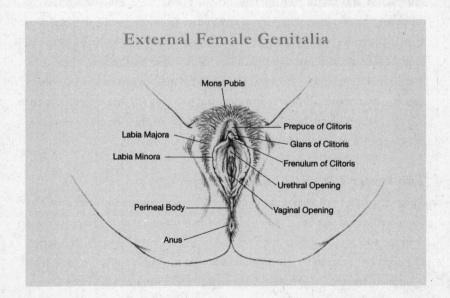

External Female Genitalia

Mons Pubis

Prepuce of Clitoris

Glans of Clitoris

Labia Majora

Labia Minora

Frenulum of Clitoris

Urethral Opening

Perineal Body

Vaginal Opening

Anus

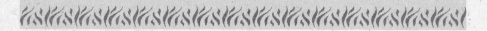

More About Pubic Hair

Somehow, finding a gray pubic hair "down there" feels worse than discovering that first one on your head. However, don't be tempted to use hair dyes and rinses on the delicate tissue of the vulva; they may cause allergic reactions, burns, and irritation. In the seventeenth and eighteenth centuries, women sometimes wore pubic wigs to replace hair lost because of age or disease. Today, unfortunately, there's nothing that can be done about pubic hair loss. Potions and lotions designed to promote scalp hair growth are not effective on the mons and may cause irritation.

pubic hair, but some scientists think that the hair may trap secretions containing pheromones, or sexual scents, that attract the opposite sex.) Over time, pubic hair may grow in thick or sparse, coarse or fine. It may be the same color and texture as the hair on your head, or it may be somewhat different. As you age, you may notice pubic hairs turn gray and begin to thin and grow sparse. Many young women intentionally shave away all their pubic hair, not just for a clean-cut bikini line, but because they say it makes their vulvas feel more sensitive. The mons contains many nerve endings, and some women find touch and massage of this area very stimulating. Others shave because they feel cleaner, or their boyfriends prefer the smooth feel of a bald vulva.

The Outer Lips (Labia majora)

The pubic hair continues down and over the *labia majora*, or outer lips. The outer surface of the labia may be smooth or wrinkled and darker in color than the surrounding skin. Don't be surprised if one of your labia is larger or longer than the other. You will notice that the inner surface of the labia is smooth, hairless, and moist because this area contains many sweat- and

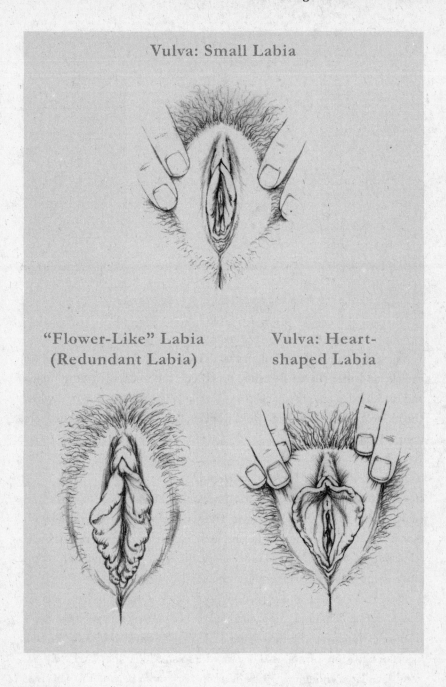

Vulva: Small Labia

"Flower-Like" Labia
(Redundant Labia)

Vulva: Heart-
shaped Labia

oil-secreting glands. (Oftentimes, my patients have mistaken the numerous large gland openings for genital warts or related conditions.)

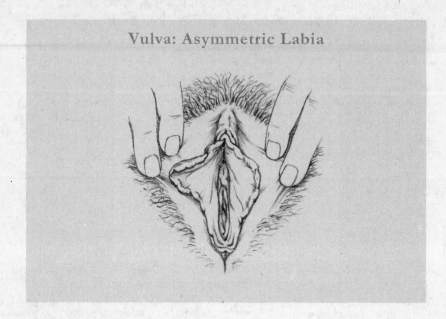

Vulva: Asymmetric Labia

These outermost lips contain fat, nerves, smooth muscle, and blood vessels, and they serve as guards, protecting the openings to the vagina and bladder. Erectile tissue deep within the labia swells with blood when you're sexually excited, and you'll notice that the lips feel full, swollen, tight, or tingly.

The Inner Lips (Labia minora)

If you spread apart your labia majora, you will notice two smooth, thin folds of skin called the *labia minora*. The sensitive inner lips are filled with blood vessels and spongy tissue and are covered with nerve endings and oil-secreting glands. Like the outer labia, the labia minora fill with blood and enlarge when you're sexually stimulated.

Don't fret if these inner lips don't look like the ones you have seen in books; the labia minora, more than any other part of our genitals, varies from one woman to the next. Your labia may be pink, burgundy, brown, black, or a mixture of colors. They may be so small that they are barely noticeable or large enough to protrude an inch or more beyond the labia majora. It's not uncommon for one to be larger than the other. They may be straight, slightly ruffled, or very wrinkled. (Contrary to the myth, neither wrinkling nor the size of your labia is increased by masturbation.) After twenty years as a gynecologist, I can tell you that no two women's labia look exactly alike. Each is unique, beautiful, and almost flowerlike. Occasionally, the labia are so large that they get snagged in underwear or pulled into the vagina during intercourse—both pretty uncomfortable occurrences. A surgical procedure can reduce the size of the labia, but it's not without risks, so it's usually performed only to reduce discomfort, not for cosmetic reasons.

The top of the labia minora come together and drape over the *glans,* or head, of the clitoris (which we'll explore a little later), forming the hood or prepuce. The hood is similar to the foreskin of an uncircumcised penis in that it protects the delicate glans. The labia meet underneath the clitoris at a point called the *frenulum,* which is intensely sensitive to stimulation. (Men have a frenulum as well, which we will discuss later.) The labia then continue toward your vagina and end just beneath the opening of your vagina.

The Pleasure Button—The Clitoris

If you look under the hood formed by the labia minora, you may be able to see a small pea or button-shaped mass, ranging in color from pink to purple to dark brown. That's your *clitoris.* If you don't see anything at first, don't worry. Sometimes it's difficult to see the clitoris even when you are sexually stimulated. Derived from the Greek word, *kleitoris,* meaning

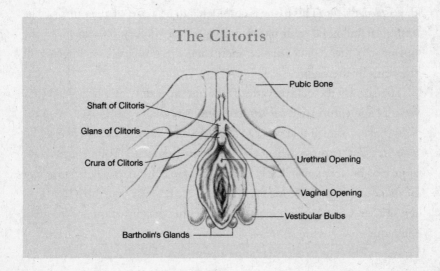

The Clitoris

Pubic Bone

Shaft of Clitoris

Glans of Clitoris

Crura of Clitoris

Urethral Opening

Vaginal Opening

Vestibular Bulbs

Bartholin's Glands

"divine and goddesslike," the clitoris has been the most ignored aspect of female sexuality in modern history. Many of us don't know where it is, how to find it, or its true size.

As a female fetus develops, the clitoris forms from the same tissue that becomes a penis in males—but it is not a "mini penis," as some people describe it. In many ways, this female organ is much more advanced! The multifunctional penis has to transport urine and sperm as well as serve as the main organ for male sexual pleasure. The clitoris is also the primary organ for female sexual pleasure—in fact, its sole purpose is pleasure.

The clitoris is much more than meets the eye. As you look at your vulva in the mirror, the clitoris may look like a tiny button of flesh hiding underneath the prepuce, but it is much more. Your clitoris is a complex, fascinating, and powerful organ.

The clitoris has a *glans, shaft,* or body, as well as *crura,* or legs. The shaft contains two *corpora cavernosa,* spongy tissue that fills with blood and increases the size of the clitoris when you become sexually stimulated. The average shaft measures 1–2 inches in length and a little over half an inch in width. But the clitoris doesn't end there. The base of the shaft attaches to the pubic bone and then divides into two crura, or legs, each measuring between 2 and 4 inches long. The crura follow and attach to the arch of the pubic bone. Extending from the base of the clitoris and lying between the crura and the labia minora are two additional masses of tissue called the *vestibular bulbs.* (This tissue is considered to be a part of the clitoris.) The vestibular bulbs fill with blood during sexual stimulation and make the opening to the vagina smaller, increasing the gripping and hugging of the penis by the vagina.

The size of the clitoris varies from one woman to the next. You may have a large clitoris that protrudes from its hood. Or you may have a clitoris that is so small that you can't easily see it (though you can usually locate it easily enough when you stimulate yourself). Your clitoris may appear to be very small if you have very large labia; if you're past the age of menopause, your clitoris may appear large because your labia have gotten smaller. Contrary to popular belief, neither masturbation nor frequent intercourse causes the clitoris to become bigger.

When it comes to pleasure and orgasm, size does not matter. With the right stimulation, even the tiniest clitoris can produce a powerful orgasm. The head of the clitoris is exquisitely sensitive, jam-packed with nerves that are larger and more numerous than the corresponding nerves in the head of the penis. The sensitivity of the clitoris also varies among women. Some women find that direct clitoral stimulation can be uncomfortable or downright painful, while others find great pleasure in prolonged stimulation of the head of the clitoris.

Pushing Your Pleasure Button

Although the clitoris is powerful, it must be handled with care. Once you learn how to stroke, massage, comfort, vibrate, rub, and love it, you are capable of experiencing divine pleasures.

Unfortunately, some people have heard that the clitoris is a small penis and think that they can treat it the same way they treat the male organ. Men may rub with gusto and suck vigorously, unaware that the pressure that works best for the penis can be too much for the average clitoris. If your sexual partner—male or female—is too energetic while manipulating the sensitive head of the clitoris, you may experience discomfort or pain. If you don't communicate clearly with your partner, your moans of pain may be mistaken for expressions of pleasure and lead to an even more intense stimulation of the clitoris. Many women tolerate pain, fake pleasure, and hope their partner will move on. Manhandling the clitoris may irritate it and leave you with a burning, swollen clitoris and labia, and difficulty walking or urinating that may last for days.

To fully enjoy the immense pleasure that the clitoris can provide—and avoid pain and discomfort—you must get to know your clitoris and what turns it on. Then you can help guide your partner in helping you experience ecstasy together. Lubricate your fingers well with a water-based vaginal lubricant or (since you're not using a condom that could be damaged by the oil) massage oil or other unscented oil. Now begin to stroke, massage, and explore your clitoris. Slowly slide your middle finger along the right side of the shaft of the clitoris and then the left. Now place your finger at the opening to your vagina and slide it up and along the head of your clitoris. Start at your mons and slide your finger down the top of the shaft, ending at the glans. Then place your index and middle finger on either

side of the shaft and labia minora. Slide both fingers down the length of
the shaft keeping contact with the sides of the shaft. As you reach the end
of the clitoris, gently squeeze the clitoris and labia between your two fingers and, maintaining the squeeze, slowly move your fingers away from
your body, bringing the clitoris and labia along for the ride.

If this is the first time you've explored your clitoris, this may not feel
pleasurable. Keep trying: Repeat these strokes and others you may come
up with, varying the amount of pressure you use and the speed of the
strokes. Discover the area of the clitoris, the type and speed of stroke, and
the amount of pressure that give you the most pleasure. Relax. As you become more comfortable with your body and your sexuality, you will be
able to discover your particular trigger points.

Once you have learned what turns you on, describe your discoveries to
your partner. Or better yet, let him watch you masturbate to learn what
makes your clitoris rise to attention. Don't be shy. Many people are quite
turned on by the sight of a woman pleasuring herself.

The Urethra

Just below the clitoris you will notice a small dimple which is the opening
to the *urethra*. The urethra is not considered a sex organ, but perhaps it
should be. Some women find the opening to the urethra to be very sensitive and stimulate it during masturbation.

Your urethra is a short tube measuring about 1½ inches long that carries urine from the bladder. It is surrounded by spongy erectile tissue that
fills with blood when you become sexually aroused. One side of your urethra lies almost directly on the front wall of your vagina. Because the
urethra and bladder are so close to your vagina, it's not unusual to feel as
if you need to urinate at the beginning of intercourse. In addition, if your
sex session is vigorous or prolonged, friction from thrusting of the penis
may cause your urethra to swell, and you may notice a temporary discomfort when you urinate after sex. Because the urethra is so short, bacteria
from your vagina or rectum can be easily pushed into your bladder during
intercourse, sometimes causing an infection.

Along the length of the urethra lie numerous small glands that open

Vulvar Self-exam

Once a month you should take a look at your vulva, just as you would do a monthly breast self-exam—and for many of the same reasons. By performing a vulvar self-exam monthly, you may be able to detect infections and vulvar cancers early. In fact, plan to do the vulvar exam at the same time you examine your breasts each month—right after your period—so you won't forget.

You'll need a mirror and a nearby light source. You can lie on the bed propped up with a pillow, sit at the edge of a chair, or stand with one leg up on a chair. With the mirror in one hand, look carefully at your vulva starting at your mons and ending at your anus. Be sure to spread the labia and pull back the hood of the clitoris, looking carefully for any new growths such as moles, bumps, or warts. If you have moles, check them regularly to see whether they grow or change color. Also note any areas of skin that have turned white, red, or a darker color. Check for any swelling, unusual discharge, or sores, and report any abnormal findings to your doctor.

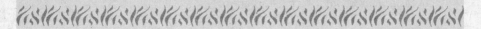

into the urethra. These *peri-urethral glands* are the female equivalent of the prostate gland in the male and, like the male counterpart, the "female prostate" may be quite sensitive to sexual stimulation, swelling with sexual arousal and perhaps releasing a fluid when some women orgasm.

The Entrance—The Introitus

The *introitus,* or opening of the vagina, lies just underneath the urethra. As you can see with your mirror, it's not a gaping hole. You may notice a very small opening when you place your finger at the opening and pull down; the opening may be larger if you've delivered a baby vaginally.

Taking Care of Your Vulva

Cleaning

༝ Wash your labia with a mild, hypoallergenic, cleansing bar or cream, or use no cleanser at all. Avoid harsh, colored, deodorant, or perfumed soaps.

༝ Make sure to spread the labia and clean the crease between the labia majora and labia minora. Thick, sticky secretions from glands in your labia can accumulate here and may not be removed by washing your vulva while in the shower. Using a soft wet cloth or the spray from a hand-held showerhead will wash away all of these secretions.

༝ To keep your clitoris clean and healthy, pull the hood of your clitoris back and, using warm water and a soft cloth, gently wipe away any secretions between the hood and the glans. Called *smegma* in men, these thick secretions contain skin cells and oil from the glands of the hood and may cause the hood to stick to the clitoris. When this happens, you may have pain during intercourse or masturbation.

༝ Wash your vulva and vaginal opening after sex. That means that if you have evening sex, you should wash before retiring for the night. Be sure to rinse away leftover whipped cream, honey, syrup, chocolate, or flavored gels if you use them during sex play. If left for long periods of time, the residue from some of these products can irritate the labia or cause infections. Besides, the natural flavor of your labia is best.

༝ Whether you are taking a bath or shower, make sure that you rinse away any soap residue from your vulva and vagina. Dry your vulva completely. A blow dryer on a cool setting can be a fun way to get rid of the moisture.

continued

❧ Do not douche. It washes away good bacteria, changes the chemical balance of the vagina, and increases your chances of an infection. It has also been shown to increase your risks of pelvic inflammatory disease (infection in your fallopian tubes).

Daily Habits

❧ Always wipe from the front to the back—from the vulva to the anus. Wiping the other way brings bacteria from the rectum into the vagina where they can cause an infection.

❧ Buy only white, unscented toilet paper—unbleached if you can find it. The dyes and fragrances in intimate paper products may be irritating.

❧ Don't bother to buy deodorant tampons, pads, and panty liners. Menstrual blood doesn't have an odor; bacteria overgrowth leads to any unpleasant smells. If you change your pads and tampons frequently you should have no odor problem.

❧ Avoid powders containing talc. Talc has been shown to increase your risk of ovarian cancer.

❧ Avoid "feminine hygiene sprays" as they may cause an allergic reaction, skin irritation, and severe inflammation of your vulva as well as increase your risk of a vaginal infection. Besides, they taste bad and may interfere with oral sex play; if your partner is allergic to the spray, the night is ruined.

❧ Before waxing, using shaving creams, or applying depilatories to remove pubic hair, apply a bit of the product to a small area of your outer labia to test for signs of irritation or allergy. Whatever hair removal method you use, be sure that none of the chemicals comes in contact with the more sensitive labia minora.

continued

❧ Don't put anything in your vagina that you would not put in your mouth. Your vagina is one of the cleanest places on your body. (It is much cleaner than your mouth.) So before you use that cucumber for sexual gratification, wash it well.

❧ Make sure that any hands that touch your vagina are clean and well manicured. Long and ragged nails are like tiny blades in the vagina.

❧ Wear all-cotton panties. Synthetic fabrics hold moisture and don't allow the vulvar skin to breathe, thus increasing your risk of an infection.

❧ Do not wear panties to bed. In fact, if you can, remove your panties and panty hose as soon as you get home.

❧ Eat a well-balanced, healthy diet. Limit your intake of simple sugars. Diets high in sugar may increase your risk of vaginal infections.

Sexual Habits

❧ Use only water-based lubricants inside your vagina. Lubricants protect a dry vagina from trauma and irritation during sex, but oil-based ones can cause a latex condom or diaphragm to weaken or tear. Oil can linger and cause infections.

❧ Do not move a penis, finger, or anything else from your rectum to your vagina without cleaning first.

❧ Use a condom to decrease your risk of sexually transmitted infections.

Troubleshooting

❧ Your labia majora and minora contain oil (*sebaceous*) glands that sometimes become clogged. When you inspect your labia with a mirror, the

continued

clogged gland will look like a typical pimple. If it becomes infected with the natural bacteria on your skin, a small, tender abscess may form. Avoid the temptation to squeeze these abcesses. Instead, soak the area with very warm moist cloths several times a day to make them disappear.

〽️ If your inner lips extend a little beyond your labia majora they may occasionally become slightly dry and irritated. Spread a thin layer of Crisco (the shortening, not the oil) on the area of labia that protrudes daily. It's a great lubricating moisturizer but should not be placed inside the vagina or used with a condom. (Oil will cause a condom to weaken and break.)

〽️ If you have severe itching of your vulva that doesn't go away, see your doctor. Itching is usually caused by an infection or skin disease but may be a sign of something more serious.

You might see tags of tissue surrounding the opening. This is tissue left from when your hymen broke. In some women, the tags aren't noticeable, but others may have large tags of tissue that seem to protrude from the vaginal opening. They alarm some women who fear that they are warts or tumors; in fact, they're perfectly normal.

You may find that the introitus is exquisitely sensitive. Use your fingers to stroke and massage this area to find your hot spots.

The Vagina

Some people view the vagina as a passive receptacle for the male penis and sperm (the word *vagina* means "sheath" in Latin) or a passageway for a baby to come through. The vagina is anything but passive, and it's more than just a hole "down there" waiting for something to come in or come out. In fact, it is a strong, luscious, expanding, complex, powerful, self-protecting,

A Rose by Any Other Name

From infancy most of us are taught to refer to our vagina as anything but vagina. It's a tee tee, pee pee, wee wee, coochie, kitty, privates, or down there. Later we hear our genitals referred to (with varying levels of explicitness) as pee hole, beaver, pocketbook, bush, muff, furburger, poontang, pookie, poonani, snatch, pussy, cunt, twat, fish box, slit, snatch, hole, crack, stink hole, love nest, playpen, baby factory, snapper, and stuff. There are probably hundreds of terms used to describe the most intimate part of our anatomy: some pet names, others derogatory terms, each suggestive word provoking different reactions from the women who hear them. Unfortunately, many of the words we use are distasteful or have negative connotations.

In some cultures, the female genitalia is honored with wonderful, creative terms. In India and Tibet, for instance, the female genitals were called the bell, cup, lotus flower or lotus of her wisdom, pleasure field of heaven, seat of pleasure, or yoni. Over the centuries, the Chinese coined dozens of terms for a woman's anatomy. Among the poetic names of the vagina were anemone of love, cinnabar crevice, conch shell, door of life, golden doorway, golden furrow, inner heart, jade gate, love grotto, mysterious valley, perfumed mouth, precious gateway, red pearl, secret cavern, and treasure house.

hormone-sensitive, ever-changing, dynamic, and fascinating organ! Even as we sleep, the vagina is on the move—contracting, lubricating, and self-cleaning.

What exactly is the vagina? The vagina lies inside your body between the bladder in the front and the rectum in the back, beginning just inside the labia minora and ending at the cervix. To truly appreciate the beauty of your vagina, you need to see it for yourself. During your next exam, ask your gynecologist to give you a mirror. After he or she inserts the speculum, position the mirror so that you can see inside, and ask your doctor to point out what's what. You can also buy your own speculum from a medical supply store and, using a mirror and light source, examine yourself inside just as you did with your vulva and external genitalia.

Your doctor uses a speculum to open the vagina because, contrary to popular belief, the vagina is not a hole, per se. It is a potential space that is typically from 2 to 2½ inches wide and ranges in length from around 3 to 6 inches, with the average vagina measuring 4.5 inches. When you aren't aroused, it's literally closed—its walls collapsed upon each other. The size of the vagina varies from one woman to another but has no relationship to the size or shape of its owner. You may be petite and your vagina long and spacious, or you may be full-figured and have a small, cozy one. (The size of your vagina doesn't have to hinder wonderful sex, either.)

The vagina has three layers. The first is similar to skin but has no hair, sweat glands, or oil-secreting glands. Warm and moist, it feels very similar to the surface of the tissue lining the inside of your mouth. Unlike your mouth, the walls of your vagina are not smooth but have many soft folds, called *rugae,* which allow it to stretch and return to its original size much like an accordion. These folds also help the pelvic muscles grip the penis during intercourse.

The second layer of the vagina, made of elastic tissue and muscle, allows the vagina to stretch—enough so that a baby can pass through—and then return to its previous size. The third layer is made of fibrous tissue and a network of blood vessels that surround the vagina. When you're sexually excited, these blood vessels swell with blood and send lots of lubricating fluids to the inside of your vagina.

Note: Be careful what you put in your vagina. Chemicals of all types may be absorbed through the layers of your vagina and into your bloodstream.

The Veil—The Hymen

If you've never had intercourse, your vagina may be guarded by the *hymen,* a term derived from the name of the ancient Greek god of marriage. Also

Does Size Matter?

Many women worry that their vaginas are either too big or too small for intercourse. Because the vagina adjusts equally well to a small or a large penis, vaginal size is usually not an obstacle to enjoyable sexual intercourse.

Things work most efficiently if your vagina and his penis size are compatible, but even if you're "short" and he is "long" or vice versa, there are techniques that have been developed over the ages to remedy this potential sexual incompatibility. The secret is to explore a variety of positions that give each person the maximum and most stimulating contact without pain or discomfort. In Chapter 4, we'll explore some of these sensuous positions.

My Vagina Is Too Small.

If you have pain as the penis enters your vagina, you may assume that your vagina is too small. The vagina is capable of stretching to accommodate any size penis. If, however, you meet a man who is extremely large, you may have some difficulty. The following tips may be helpful if you fear that your vagina is too small:

≫ Make sure that you are relaxed. Tense muscles can interfere with the ability of the vagina to stretch. You may also have difficulty lubricating adequately.

≫ Spend lots of time on foreplay. As you become more aroused, your vagina not only becomes wet but also increases in length and width.

≫ Use lubricants even if you feel that you are moist. Apply generously to the penis and the opening of your vagina.

≫ Go slowly to allow your vagina time to stretch over the penis.

continued

✺ Choose positions that limit the depth of penetration. Lie on the bottom with your legs straight. This position will allow your inner thighs and labia to add length to your vagina. You might also try side-to-side positions. The woman-on-top positions allow you to control how deeply the penis penetrates.

✺ If you are past the age of menopause and are not taking hormones, you may have dryness and shortening of your vagina. Estrogen hormones and moisturizers may help. Penis-shaped dilators (your doctor can write a prescription) may be used to stretch the vagina if needed.

✺ Discuss your concerns with your doctor or midwife.

My Vagina Is Too Big.

After having a baby make its way through your vagina, you may worry that it will forever be too large for satisfying sex. Occasionally men complain that the vagina seems too large and loose after childbirth. Many have bought into the myth that the vagina is never quite as tight or enjoyable after a baby passes through. In fact, the vagina does stretch during vaginal childbirth, but within several months it returns almost to the size it was prior to delivery.

When repairing an *episiotomy* (the cut made in the perineum as the baby is delivered) after childbirth, some gynecologists will place a large stitch at the opening of the vagina. Called the "husband's stitch," this suture makes the opening of the vagina smaller and is supposed to increase the pleasure of the male partner when sex resumes. But women who receive the stitch may find that sex in the months following childbirth may be painful.

Better to forego the stitch and look for ways to approach sex that are comfortable and pleasurable for both partners. If you feel less friction or fullness during sex, try:

continued

❧ *Kegel exercises.* Strengthening the muscles that surround the vagina will make the vagina feel tighter and will help you "grip" his penis during intercourse (see the Kegel description on page 182).

❧ *New positions.* Any position in which you keep your legs straight and closed will increase the tension within the vaginal walls. You can use the strength of your inner thigh muscles to help massage and maneuver the penis and maximize pleasure for both of you. If you choose the missionary position, for example, you lie on the bottom with your legs extended straight, and he lies on top with his legs either straight or straddling yours. You can get the same result if you're on top or you are both on your sides. If your vagina is long, pull your knees up against your chest while in the missionary position to shorten the vagina and allow deeper penetration.

❧ *Pelvic movements.* Rather than moving in and out like a piston, move your lower body in circular or side-to-side motions to increase contact between the penis and the vaginal walls.

❧ *Surgery.* I generally do not recommend surgery to tighten the vagina, especially if a woman requests this procedure solely because of complaints of her male partner. (Having surgery will not necessarily make the relationship with a disgruntled partner any better.) There are a few women, however, who experience serious tears of the vagina or the perineum, or injuries to the muscles of the pelvic floor during childbirth. A procedure called *perineoplasty,* or vaginal repair, can correct defects in the muscle of the pelvic floor and remove excess vaginal tissue—and, for some women, improve their enjoyment of sex.

known as the "veil of the temple," the hymen is delicate vaginal tissue that rims the vaginal opening without completely covering it. You can insert a tampon or be examined with a small speculum or finger without tearing the hymen.

For centuries, alum and other astringent chemicals have been used by women to dry out and shrink the size of their vaginas prior to intercourse. In parts of Africa, women use herbs and traditional concoctions to the same effect. The resulting dryness and tightness increase the friction felt by the male, making his experience more enjoyable. The experiences of the women, however, may have been quite uncomfortable due to increased bruising, swelling, abrasions, and increased infections of the vagina.

The hymen usually has one opening but occasionally may have two or more. The hymen is said to be *imperforate* and abnormal if it completely covers the opening to the vagina. A girl with this condition will need surgery during puberty to open the hymen and allow menstrual blood to flow out.

The first sexual intercourse will probably cause small tears in the hymen and you might see a small amount of blood, but not always. A virgin might not bleed when she is "deflowered" if her hymen stretches rather than tears during intercourse. Too, some women are born with only a very small rim of hymenal tissue, and some athletic women may "break" their hymens through their participation in sports. The lack of blood does not make them any less a virgin. In some cultures, however, this blood is so important in proving virginity that the stained wedding-night sheets may even be displayed for the community to see. Women have lost their lives if they failed to bleed. For this reason, women who are concerned that they might not bleed have devised ingenious ways to satisfy their mates. In Sudan, some women have placed tiny bags containing chicken blood into their vaginas prior to intercourse. In other countries, congealed balls of sheep blood have served the same purpose. Scheduling your wedding night to coincide with your menses assures a blood-stained sheet. And plastic surgeons have perfected a surgical method to re-create the hymen.

Vaginal Secretions

Vaginal secretions are normal and important for the health of your vagina. Without secretions, the delicate tissues of your vagina would dry out. Normal vaginal secretions are made up of a complex mixture of cells that are shed from the walls of the vagina; healthy vaginal bacteria; vaginal fluid; vulvar secretions from sebaceous glands, sweat, Bartholin's glands; and a small amount of fluid from the uterus and fallopian tubes. These secretions are a nutritious mix of carbohydrates, amino acids, proteins, and acids produced by the abundant lactobacilli bacteria. They're not only normal but also important in keeping your vagina moist and healthy.

The vagina is a self-cleansing organ. You may notice thick, white secretions that coat your panties at the end of the day, or clumps of thick mucus or cottage cheese–like emissions. This may go one for a few days or weeks, but it's normal and shouldn't be confused with abnormal vaginal discharge caused by an infection and usually accompanied by itching, burning, or a foul odor.

The amount and consistency of normal vaginal secretions vary from one woman to the next. Some women produce copious amounts of vaginal fluids—enough to leave them feeling wet at the end of the day. If there is no burning, itching, or foul odor, and a gynecological exam and vaginal cultures are normal, the heavy secretions are most likely normal for you. Try wearing unscented panty liners and changing them frequently during the day to keep the vulva dry and to avoid irritation.

Other women find that their vaginal secretions are less than adequate, leaving them with a scratchy, sometimes burning sensation. Birth control pills, breast feeding, menopause, medications, or chronic douching may be the culprit. Vaginal moisturizers and water-soluble personal lubricants may help.

The amount, color, and texture of vaginal secretions may change during the month. Just before you ovulate, you may notice more clear, stringy, mucouslike secretions that some women describe as slimy like egg whites. After ovulation, the secretions may become thick, sticky, or clumpy and white. Vaginal secretions may yellow when dry. (You may also notice yellow stains in your panties after washing them. This happens when your normal acidic secretions react with detergents. It's not an indication of an infection.)

How to Tell When Something Is Wrong

Though vaginal secretions are normal, sometimes a change in your secretions is a sign that something may be wrong. Look out for the following:

Unusual color. Normal secretions are clear or white. A change may represent an infection. Green discharge usually indicates a bacterial infection. A yellow discharge may represent a sexually transmitted infection such as gonorrhea, chlamydia, or another bacterial infection. And if you notice a heavy yellow discharge you should see your health-care provider for cultures. Brown or pink discharge may be normal if it occurs just before or just at the end of your period, but if you see it at other times, it may be a sign of a problem.

Odor. Normal vaginal odor is musky and clean. If your vaginal odor becomes foul, it may indicate that you have an infection. The most common infection to cause an offensive odor is *bacterial vaginosis* (discussed later), though any infection can make your vaginal scent unpleasant. Anything that is left in the vagina too long—a tampon or diaphragm that is forgotten or a condom that is lost during intercourse, for example—can cause a foul vaginal discharge and produce a wicked odor.

Itching or burning. We all have occasional episodes of itching. If a few scratches offer relief, it's most likely not significant. More severe or unrelenting itching or burning of the vulva can be signs of an infection. The most common culprits are trichomonas and yeast; other causes include scabies (also known as "crabs"), allergic reactions, and dermatitis. Dryness of the vagina, herpes, and human papilloma virus infections may also cause a combination of itching and burning.

continued

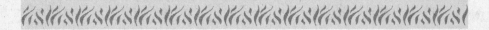

🌿 *Profuse, watery discharge.* Women with fibroids, cervical infections, or fallopian tube disease may have this symptom. After menopause, thinning of the walls of the vagina may cause the vagina to "weep" and produce a clear, watery discharge. And you may notice watery secretions up to 24 hours after intercourse.

When you become sexually aroused, your vagina produces clear secretions—the lubrication that makes it easier to penetrate the vagina during intercourse or manual sex play. The blood flowing to the walls of your vagina increases during arousal, and as the vessels surrounding your vagina become more congested, fluid is forced through your vaginal walls. At first the fluid looks like small beads of sweat on the vaginal walls, but the more aroused you become, the more fluid presses through, coating your vagina with the slippery fluid. The amount of lubrication that you produce may not be the same as someone else, and it may vary from one experience to the next or over time.

Vaginal Odors

No one seems to know who started the myth that the vagina smells like fish, but everybody seems to believe it. We're taught early on, either verbally or nonverbally, that our vaginas smell bad. The advertising media have capitalized on our insecurity about how we smell and convinced us that our natural scent is unpleasant and should be destroyed, deodorized, sanitized, suppressed, masked, and replaced with the scent of flowers. Pharmacies sell sprays, soaps, powders, creams, deodorants, scented sanitary pads and tampons, all meant to rid us of our natural female scent.

The natural odor of the vagina can best be described as a pleasant musky scent, though each woman has her own "signature" scent. Normal vaginal scents are considered quite sexually stimulating by our sexual partners. Indeed some women have found that when they spread their vaginal

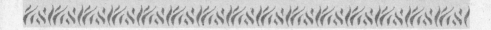

A Telltale Scent?

Some of my patients have complained of a "semenlike" vaginal odor the day after intercourse without a condom. Their greatest fear is that others will perceive the telltale odor. The slightest glance of a colleague may be interpreted as an "I know what you did last night" look. Semen has a distinctive scent, particularly when blended with your vaginal secretions, and may drip for hours after intercourse. But it's unlikely that others are aware of any odor.

Don't be tempted to douche. Instead, place a tampon in the vagina after bathing. The remaining semen will be absorbed, and the tampon can be removed in a couple of hours.

secretions on their breasts prior to intimate contact, their male partners have larger and harder erections.

It's important that you become familiar with your unique scent in order to appreciate the power that it holds and to make it easier for you to detect vaginal infections. To begin to become more familiar with your unique scent, place a well-washed finger (carefully trim your fingernails) into your vagina as far as feels comfortable for you; don't allow your finger to touch your vulva. Remove your finger, wave it about 3 inches in front of your nose, breathe deeply. That's your own personal fragrance.

Your vaginal odor can be affected by what you eat, drink, or smoke. A diet high in meat products, garlic, onions, spicy food, and alcohol can change the character and intensity of your odor. Some say that the resulting secretions aren't as sweet in smell or taste. Likewise, smoking cigarettes or marijuana can play havoc on your natural aroma, as can some medications and hormones. Birth control pills tend to decrease your vaginal scent.

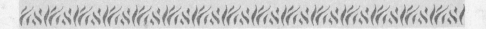

Douching

A healthy vagina does a very good job of cleansing itself; *douching* (flushing out the vagina with water or a combination of water and other cleansing agents) can interfere with its natural process, doing more harm than good. Douching, even with a mild product, can dry and injure the delicate lining of the vagina and can increase your risk of infection by changing the natural environment of the vagina, thereby reducing its acidity and leaving the vagina susceptible to infection. In addition, you may put yourself more at risk of pelvic inflammatory disease (PID). Douching may also mask a more serious infection and delay its appropriate treatment.

If you feel that you absolutely must douche, use a disposable, mild, unscented water-and-vinegar douche. In general, I suggest that you avoid douching unless prescribed by your doctor for a specific problem.

The scent of your vagina also changes during your monthly menstrual cycle. The most pleasant scent occurs during the period surrounding ovulation, or the middle of your cycle. (It makes biological sense, because this is the time the woman's body is fertile and wants to attract a partner to fertilize those eggs.) Sometimes at the end of your period, the flow of blood slows down to a small slow trickle and is caught in the many folds of the vagina. The bacteria that normally live in the vagina may interact with the blood and produce an unpleasant odor.

You might notice that the scent of your vagina changes after your partner ejaculates in your vagina—and this scent may be different with each man that you have sex with. The semen of a particular man may produce a foul odor when mixed with your vaginal secretions. And a weekend of multiple episodes of intercourse may leave your vagina with a less-than-pleasant odor.

Most of the odor that we perceive when we remove our panties does not actually come from the vagina but from the vulva. The mons and labia majora are covered with hair as well as lots of sweat- and oil-secreting glands; the labia minora and clitoral hood also contain oil glands. The oil on the skin, pubic hair, and clothing hold in the moisture and create a warm, damp environment that's a great breeding ground for the natural bacteria that we all have on our skin and genitals, bacteria that, when it multiplies, produces an unpleasant odor. When we wear panties, panty hose, and pants (and we often wear them all at the same time), we are inviting a problem. If you wear panty hose, choose brands with a cotton crotch and don't wear panties with them. Or skip panty hose and pull on stockings and garter belt, thigh highs, or socks. And remember, stress can also cause increased sweating in your vulva.

Thick, oily smegma may accumulate between the folds of your labia and under the hood of your clitoris, places that also serve as wonderful playgrounds for odor-causing bacteria. Wash well between the folds of the labia and pubic area each day, keeping the vulva as dry as possible, and wear clothes that allow your skin to breathe. If you are very concerned about your odor, you can carry unscented diaper wipes and use them to clean your vulva and perineum after every trip to the bathroom. (To avoid irritation, make sure they're scent and alcohol free.) If you carry a large purse, another option is to carry a small plastic bottle with a squirt top. You can fill it with warm water and spray your vulva before you wipe. Of course, if a bidet is available, that's an even better solution.

Vaginal Sensations

Another myth about the vagina is that it contains few nerve endings and thus has no feeling. Sadly, this one has been passed on from one generation of doctors to the next. During my residency, we were told that you could biopsy the vagina without anesthesia. No one seemed to question why the women screamed as the tiny pieces of flesh were removed.

The person who first described the vagina as an "insensitive" organ obviously didn't have one. Today we know that the vagina is, in fact, well endowed with nerves and feelings. The opening of the vagina, the front wall, and all around the lower third of it tend to be the most sensitive. Some women may find the back wall or the top of the vagina near the cervix to be quite sensitive as well.

Some, though not all women, have an area on the front wall of the vagina that is especially sensitive to stimulation. Located on the front vaginal wall about midway up the vagina from the opening, this area was described in 1950 by German gynecologist Dr. Ernst Grafenberg, hence its name: the G-spot. Though Dr. Grafenberg has been credited with the discovery of this sensitive area, ancient Indian and Chinese writings also describe what they called the "sacred spot." This area of the vagina was thought to hold the key to female sexual pleasure; proper stimulation could lead not only to powerful orgasms, but to female ejaculation as well. Today, the G-spot is thought to be the equivalent of the prostate gland in men, and when you stimulate this area—a bumpy region the size of a bean—it swells and, indeed, may bring some women to orgasm.

To discover this secret spot, use a clean, lubricated, well-manicured finger. Insert it carefully into the vagina, feeling the warmth, softness, and moisture of the vaginal walls. Move your finger farther in until you touch something that feels like the tip of your nose. That's your cervix. (You may need to squat to get your finger far enough into your vagina.) Now, keeping your finger inside, slide your fingertips along the front wall until you're halfway between your vaginal opening and your cervix. Feel around for a small bumpy patch of tissue. Now gently massage this area as you curl your fingers in a beckoning, "come here" motion. Initially, you may feel like you need to urinate, but as you continue the massage, you may find that the area begins to swell and feel warm and wonderful. If it feels good, enjoy it.

Remember, however, that not all women find stimulation of this area pleasurable. If all you feel is numbness, don't rub yourself raw; take a break and try again another time. Search for other sensitive areas by moving your finger around the entire surface of your vagina in and out and in small circles, exploring around all sides of your cervix, the top of the vagina, then the back wall, the sides, and finally the sensitive tissue at the opening. Make a mental note of the areas that brought you the most pleasure. Don't become discouraged if you don't find a pleasurable spot the first time you explore your vagina. It sometimes takes multiple explorations before treasure is found—and locating it can be a ton of fun.

Vaginal Sounds

Sometimes when you prop your hips on pillows during sex or assume a position that raises your pelvis high, air gets sucked into the vagina and trapped there as the top portion of your vagina expands. (Similarly, standing on your head or assuming yoga and exercise positions that significantly raise your pelvis may have the same effect.) If you lower your pelvis or if he's thrusting vigorously during sex, you may hear a loud "fartlike" sound from your vagina. There's no reason to be embarrassed; the sound is normal, it's not gas and it has no odor.

You may sometimes notice a "swishing" sound as the thrusting and other motions of intercourse move your vaginal secretions around. This, too, is normal. Don't worry that your vagina is too big or too wet. In fact, enjoy your juicy sounds; many people find these sounds very arousing.

Vaginal Taste

Yes, vaginal secretions can stimulate the taste buds, too, just like any other delicious nectar. As with scent, each woman is endowed with her own flavor, a taste that may range from sweet to slightly salty and may change throughout the month. At times, vaginal fluids may have no taste at all; at other times the taste of your secretions may be affected by medications and what you eat, drink, or smoke. Diets high in animal protein and dairy products, as well as excessive consumption of alcohol, nicotine, caffeine, and marijuana may leave a bad taste in your (or his/her) mouth. For better-tasting juices, eat plenty of fruits, vegetables, and whole grains. But avoid asparagus! This stalky vegetable can cause the vaginal fluids to have a foul taste and smell.

Before you ask someone else to appreciate your particular "flavor," you might want to learn to appreciate it yourself. Place a clean, well-manicured finger into your vagina, then taste the fluids you find there. Before you think "Yuck!" remember that your vagina is one of the cleanest parts of your body—much cleaner than your mouth. You will ingest more germs during a passionate kiss than you will from taste-testing your own vaginal juices.

Vaginal Infections

The normal vagina is highly acidic and contains millions of bacteria living harmoniously inside your body. One species of bacteria, the *lactobacilli,* produces hydrogen peroxide that keeps the other bacteria in check and prevents their overgrowth. But occasionally, something goes awry and yeast or bacteria overgrow, causing an infection, or *vaginitis.* Stress, an unhealthy diet, medical problems such as diabetes, and taking antibiotics can increase the likelihood of having some types of vaginitis. Most women will have at least one episode of vaginal infection during their lifetime.

Bacterial Vaginosis (BV)

The most common type of vaginal infection is *bacterial vaginosis.* Also known as *nonspecific vaginitis,* it's caused by bacteria (usually *Gardnerella vaginalis* and other anaerobic bacteria) that normally live in the vagina in small numbers but that have multiplied and outgrown the good bacteria. The infection causes a thin, gray or green discharge that has a foul fishy odor that typically becomes even worse during menstruation or when the vaginal secretions mix with semen. Symptoms, if there are any, include vaginal itching and burning. Bacterial vaginosis can be treated with antibiotic tablets or vaginal cream for five to seven days. BV isn't considered a sexually transmitted infection, but if you have recurrent infections your partner may need to be treated.

Yeast Infection

Candidiasis, or yeast infection, is most commonly caused by *Candida albicans,* a fungus normally found in small numbers in the vagina, though other types of fungi can also be responsible. Yeast infections cause severe itching and/or burning of the vulva and vagina. We usually think of the discharge caused by yeast as thick and curdlike, similar to cottage cheese. However the discharge may be sparse and thin. Sometimes all you see is redness and swelling of the vulva and vagina. (Thick, white discharge alone doesn't mean you have a yeast infection.)

Yeast infections are very common and may be triggered by stress, a diet high in sugars and carbohydrates, antibiotics, birth control pills, pregnancy, or tight-fitting clothing. Or you may get one for no reason at all. Treatments include vaginal creams, tablets, or suppositories containing antifungal agents that you use for one to seven days. Be sure that you use the medications in your vagina as well as on your vulva as both are usually infected at the same time with yeast.

If you have been diagnosed with a yeast infection in the past, and you are sure that you have a recurrence rather than something more serious, you can buy yeast-curing creams and suppositories over the counter. But if you are not sure that your symptoms are caused by yeast, you should see your health-care provider. A physician may sometimes prescribe an oral tablet instead of the creams.

If you have frequent yeast infections try eating a cup of plain yogurt containing *Lactobacillus acidophilus* every day. (You will have to check the label to be sure that the brand you buy contains the right culture.) Daily supplements of acidophilus and garlic tablets may also help fend off vaginal infections.

Sexual intercourse while you have a yeast infection can be very painful, and, because semen is alkaline, having sex without a condom during a yeast episode will make it easier for the yeast to grow and make the infection worse. If you have oral sex, your partner may complain that your vaginal secretions have a sour taste and odor. Don't have sex while you're suffering with a yeast infection. (If you simply can't resist having intercourse, use a condom and place the medication in your vagina after sex.) A yeast infection is not considered a sexually transmitted infection though your partner may need to be treated if you have frequent, recurrent infections.

Trichomoniasis

Trichomoniasis is caused by a parasite called trichomonas that may be transmitted by sexual or, in a few cases, nonsexual means. You may notice severe itching of the vulva and vagina as well as a foul-smelling discharge that's thin, watery, frothy, and may be yellow, green, or gray. Sometimes you may have no symptoms at all.

Trichomoniasis infection is treated with a one-day course of antibiotics, though sometimes a longer course is necessary. Because trichomoniasis infection can be transmitted during intercourse, your sex partner must be treated.

If your doctor diagnoses a vaginal infection, it's very important that you complete the entire course of medication. You may feel better within hours of starting the treatment, but if you stop taking the medication too soon you may have a recurrence of the infection. Having intercourse while you have a vaginal infection may cause severe burning or irritation, so you may want to abstain. Ask your doctor if intercourse is advisable while being treated for the infection.

Your Internal Sex Organs

The Cervix

If you put your finger all the way into your vagina, reaching as far up as you can, you'll feel the cervix, firm and rounded, almost like the tip of your nose. The *cervix,* the lower part of the uterus, serves as an entrance for sperm and the exit for menstrual blood, secretions, and babies. Because for so long, scientists reported that the cervix had no nerve endings and lacked sensation, many people don't realize that some women find stimulation of the cervix to be highly pleasurable. A few can reach orgasm by stimulation of the cervix alone.

Cells inside the cervix secrete mucus that, just prior to ovulation, is abundant, thin, clear, and slimy. This mucus makes it easier for sperm to swim up your cervix and into your uterus during your most fertile days. After ovulation, the mucus decreases and becomes thicker.

You or your partner may sometimes notice a small bump (or bumps) on your cervix when you touch it. These *Nabothian cysts* occur when mucous-secreting cells on the cervix become blocked. Most are the size of a small green pea but may be larger or smaller. They're common, benign, don't cause problems, and don't need treatment.

To make sure that you keep your cervix healthy, see your doctor or midwife for a pap smear every year. Schedule your appointment for one to two

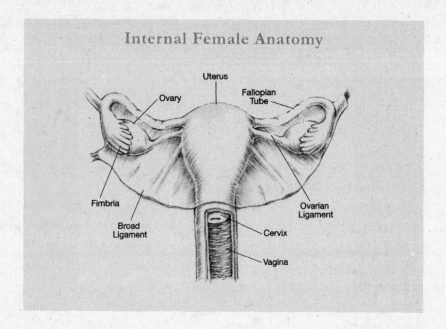

Internal Female Anatomy

Uterus

Ovary

Fallopian Tube

Fimbria

Ovarian Ligament

Broad Ligament

Cervix

Vagina

weeks after your period ends. And don't douche, use vaginal medications, or have intercourse for 48 hours prior to your exam.

The Uterus

The uterus looks like an upside-down pear that's usually about the size of your fist, though it may be smaller if you are menopausal, or larger if you have had several children. A thin layer of moist tissue covers the uterus.

Every month the inside layer of the uterus, the *endometrium,* becomes thick and plush. If you become pregnant, the fertilized egg attaches to the soft tissue inside your uterus—and stays there. If you don't become pregnant, the tissue sloughs off as menstrual blood. If you become pregnant, a thick layer of muscle that surrounds the endometrium stretches as the baby grows, contracts when you go into labor, and returns to its previous size after childbirth.

Some physicians don't view the healthy uterus as important in a woman's sexual functioning. But some women are rather acutely aware of contractions of the uterus during orgasm, and some have noted a decrease in the intensity of orgasm after a hysterectomy.

The Fallopian Tubes

You have two fallopian tubes, each about 4 inches long, which extend from both sides of your uterus. When an egg is released from your ovary, it travels down the fallopian tube toward the uterus. If sperm are swimming around there, they may fertilize the egg, which then continues its trip to the uterus to be implanted.

Sometimes, however, the fallopian tubes may become infected and damaged by sexually transmitted diseases such as chlamydia. Infection of the fallopian tubes, called *salpingitis,* is also more common if you use an IUD for contraception and have multiple sex partners. Salpingitis causes sex to be intensely painful.

The Ovaries

Attached to each side of your uterus by ligaments is an almond-sized ovary, both of which produce the female hormones *estrogen* and *progesterone* as well as a small amount of the male hormone *testosterone*. All of these hormones are important to our sexual health, as we will discuss later.

When you are born, these little ovaries each contain about 400,000 eggs, and your body doesn't produce any more during your lifetime. Each month that you ovulate, one egg is released for possible fertilization. That means that approximately 300–400 eggs are released during your reproductive lifetime.

Chapter 2

Erogenous Zones

When we think of sex, we usually think of the genitals, and when we talk about sex, we're generally discussing intercourse. So when we're speaking of pleasing a lover sexually, we generally think of how we will stimulate the person's vital sexual organs—the areas we know will have a sexual response. But sex is so much more than that.

Instead of thinking only of the genitals when we think of turning our partner (or ourselves) on, we should think of how to make sex a total body experience. Too often we rush to the genitals and neglect the other sensual, sensitive, and pleasurable body parts. For a truly satisfying sex life, take the time to discover the location of your erogenous zones and those of your partner. Because every woman (and man) is different, what may be thrilling to you may not be to your partner. What worked for one lover may not do anything for another. That just means that you and your lover have dozens of square inches of skin and other body parts to touch and explore.

Perineum and Anus

Just beyond the vaginal opening is the anus, the opening to the rectum and exit for the bowels. The anus has hundreds of nerves, and some women find stroking this area quite arousing. In fact, the anus is one of the most sensitive areas of your body. Gently stroking the skin surrounding the anus with a feather, finger, or tongue can send some women over the edge. You may also enjoy the sensations created when a finger is slowly inserted into your anus. (The anus does not produce its own lubrication so you need a lubricant or oil to ease the insertion of a finger.) Also be sure anything that goes from anus to vagina (finger, sex toy) is washed to avoid the spread of bacteria.

If you take your mirror and look just past the opening of your vagina at the area between it and the anus, you'll be looking at the perineum, an area that some women also find quite sensitive to touch and pressure. Massaging this area with warm oil can be intensely pleasurable.

Skin

Any body part covered in skin has the potential to be an erogenous zone. In particular, the places near the sexual organs and those areas that have many nerve endings and are especially ticklish or sensitive can be erogenous zones.

For wonderful skin-to-skin contact, make sure you keep your skin smooth and soft. When you bathe, use a loofa or other scrubber to buff your skin to make it softer and more sensitive to being touched. Use oils and lotions after you bathe or at other times during the day to make your skin extra soft.

Be careful about touching areas of broken skin. Skin that is raw and inflamed will become sore and tender when stroked, killing what should be a sensual experience.

Ears

Ears are sensory organs and respond to sensual pleasures. You may find soft romantic whispers in your ears to be highly arousing—the bursts of soft breath as your lover murmurs sweet nothings can tickle and thrill your ears. Many people enjoy feeling the exploration of a warm, moist tongue along the ear's many winding curves, or gentle nibbling and sucking of earlobes.

Neck

The neck is sensitive, complex, curvy, and inviting. Blowing warm air, placing light kisses, or stroking with fingers or tongue here can be a real turn-on. The throat and the little dimple between the collarbones, especially in men, is sensitive and sensual. Start at the collarbone and kiss your way up to the chin using your mouth or fingers. Or simply nuzzle into your partner's neck.

Hair

Running your fingers through your lover's hair has always been considered erotic. Adding a scalp massage helps to warm things up. Give special attention to the hairline.

Mouth

A good kisser can nearly bring you to orgasm, so surely the mouth qualifies as an erogenous zone. Mouths are wet, soft, warm, and full of nerve endings—much like the genitals—so they can turn you on in similar ways. Your lips and tongue are two of the most sensitive areas of your body.

Back

You may never have thought of your back as erotic, but it is packed with nerve endings and can provide immense sexual pleasure. For some, a back

rub is the prelude to lovemaking; a good massage can make you more relaxed and receptive to sex play. Light strokes, kisses, and tongue play along
your spine can send sensuous shivers through your body. The small trian-
gle that's formed where your spine meets your buttocks is a very sensitive
spot in many people (male and female), so you might want to spend some
time kissing and rubbing this area.

Navel

Kissing and licking the navel can be very arousing. This little button looks
innocent enough, but the sensitive umbilicus can really pack a wallop. Some
may even find it extremely ticklish, which can add to the playfulness of sex.

Some men find the area just below the navel, the lower abdomen, to be
especially sensitive. Stroking this area may give him a wonderful sensation.

Thighs

The inner thigh is soft, sensitive, and, for some people, ticklish. It is the
entryway to the genitals, so being touched there can be exciting because it
creates a sense of anticipation that the lover's hands (or kisses) will wander
upward. The place where the inner thigh meets the pubic area is an especially sensitive area for some. Try massaging, sucking, and stroking here.

Buttocks

Butts are sexy. These muscles are the main movers and shakers of your
pelvis during lovemaking, and because the buttocks are richly supplied
with nerve endings, squeezing, stroking, massaging, and kissing them can
be highly arousing. The crease where the buttocks meet the upper thighs
may be particularly sensitive.

Feet and Toes

The feet and toes can be very sensitive to touch and massage. Imagine
your lover taking your feet in his hands, pouring warm oil over them, and

giving them a gentle massage. Imagine that he's stroking the soles of your feet, kissing and sucking your toes. Try taking turns with your lover, giving such attention to each other's feet.

Hands

It is very romantic to have a man kiss your hand. How sexy if he kisses or tickles your palm. How hungry he is for you if he sucks your fingertips or nibbles the inside of your wrist or carries his kisses up your arm to the sensitive curve of your elbow. Hands are wonderfully sensitive—to touch with or to be touched.

Breasts

A major part of lovemaking and sexual play, the breasts are often considered much more than an erogenous zone. There are almost as many different kinds of breasts as there are women—and often we have a love/hate relationship with our bosoms. Few of us are completely happy with them. We think they're too small or too large; ride too high or hang too low; are too sensitive to touch or not sensitive enough. The nipples are too large, too small, turn too far in, stick too far out, or have too much hair around them. We fear that they will wither and sag as we age. And we wonder if our partners will find them attractive. Breasts not only vary in size, shape, firmness, and sensitivity from one woman to another, they may also change over a woman's lifetime. They're just a pair of simple mounds of tissue, but we experience a great deal of angst about our mammary glands.

In truth, though we spend so much time thinking about whether or not we have a perfect-looking pair, breasts are first and foremost functional organs: We have them so that we can feed our offspring. Eighty percent of a woman's breast is fat and connective tissue; the rest is made of glands and ducts. The glands—you have 12–20 groups of them—produce milk that is then transported through the ducts to your nipple and flows out as nourishment for an infant.

There are many countries in the world where women walk around bare breasted—absolutely un-self-conscious—because breasts are simply

Internal Breast

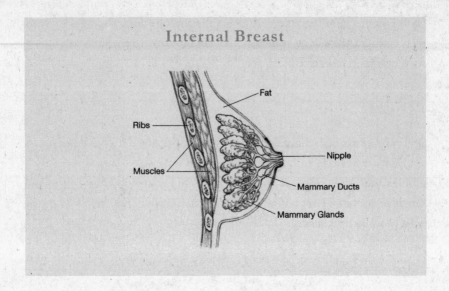

functional body parts, no sexier than a foot or a hand. In the West, the breast is also a sexual organ—at least for some women. Some women don't get any sexual pleasure from having their nipples touched or tweaked, and may even find it a turn-off. Every woman will likely have "hands-off-the-breasts" days. At times in your life when you experience changes in hormone levels (just before or during your period, during the first days of pregnancy, or as you enter menopause) your breasts may be so tender that the thought of someone touching them makes you cringe.

However, many women find it very pleasing to have their breasts touched, stroked, massaged, and sucked. The nipple—a sensitive little button of flesh that, when manipulated, can bring some women to orgasm—contains hundreds of nerves as well as smooth muscle that contracts when you are sexually aroused, causing the nipple to become hard and erect.

Contrary to popular myths, large breasts do not respond better sexually than small ones, and large-busted women don't necessarily enjoy or crave sex more than women with small breasts. But so much emphasis has been placed on breast size that some women can't fully enjoy sex because they're concerned that their breasts don't measure up. That insecurity leads many women to look for methods to make their breasts larger. If that's your goal,

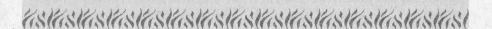

If your partner is a champion breast sucker, you may notice a small amount of milky discharge from your breasts if you squeeze your nipples. Because your body can't differentiate between the urgent sucking of a hungry baby and a horny adult, your brain responds by secreting *prolactin,* the hormone that makes milk. Birth control pills, narcotics, and other medications can also cause a milky discharge. However, any discharge from your breasts should be evaluated by your doctor to make sure there is nothing more serious happening.

You may also notice small bumps surrounding your nipple. These are oil-secreting glands that help keep the nipples moist and lubricated, but they may sometimes become clogged like a pimple. Don't squeeze them! Use warm cloths as compresses and wait for them to soften and disappear naturally. If this method doesn't seem to work after several days, or the bumps become red and painful, see your doctor.

know that you can't increase your breast size with any of the numerous suction devices and lotions advertised in magazines and on the Internet. Birth control pills will sometimes make breasts a little bigger, and bulking up your *pectoralis major muscles* (the chest muscles directly underneath your breasts) through weight training will sometimes make the bustline appear bigger. Of course your breasts can also be enlarged (or reduced in size) by plastic surgery. But be aware that surgery can sometimes change the sensitivity and sexual response of your breasts and nipples. Be sure to discuss all of the pros and cons of breast surgery with your doctor.

Breast Self-Exam

Every year, approximately 184,000 women are diagnosed with breast cancer. When you're between thirty-five and forty years old, your doctor will likely suggest that you have a mammogram, but even before then, you should check your breasts monthly looking for changes in the breast tissue. It's the most effective way to detect a possible abnormality early.

The best time to perform the exam is three or four days after your period ends. Your hormone levels are lower and the breasts are less tender and "lumpy" feeling. If you don't have periods, choose the first of each month or any other date that you will find easy to remember.

Begin your exam by standing in front of a mirror in a well-lit room. With your hands at your side, look at your breasts with an eye for anything that seems unusual. It is normal for one breast to be slightly larger than the other. Look for dimpling, puckering, or areas of the skin that look similar to orange peel and note any redness or swelling. Look at your nipples, paying attention to any areas that seem to be pulled in or pushed out. Continuing to observe your breasts, raise your arms above your head. Now bring your hands down and press them into your hips, contracting your chest muscles. Again look for changes in the skin or nipples of your breasts. Compare the two breasts, looking for asymmetry.

Next, lie flat on your back, placing a small pillow just under your right shoulder and raise your right arm above your head. This "spreads" your breast over a wider area of your chest and makes the exam easier. Begin the exam under your arm. Using the flat part of the fingers of your left hand, make small circular motions while pressing your breast tissue against your chest wall. Look for lumps, bumps, thickening, or areas that have changed since your last exam. Continue the circular motions as you move in closer to your nipple. Make several complete circles around the breast, making sure that you haven't missed a single spot. Press your nipple against your chest wall. Now gently squeeze the nipple and look for any discharge. Repeat all of the steps on the left side.

You can also do this exam while you're standing in the shower; some women find the exam much easier when their hands glide across their slippery wet skin. Report any suspicious findings to your doctor.

Chapter 3

His Body: Male Sexual Anatomy

A woman's sexual satisfaction may be enhanced by her knowledge of male anatomy. If you have sex with men, there are many reasons to learn everything you can about their bodies. Learning to appreciate the beauty of your partner's anatomy will allow you to feel more comfortable and less inhibited during sex. Your understanding of how his sexual anatomy works will be invaluable not only in pleasing him, but the more you know and understand what makes him tick will help you achieve the most pleasure in your sexual encounters.

Penis

Some women have told me that they find the male genitals to be "ugly" and "repulsive." However, other than the fact that yours is internal and his is external, the male and female sex organs are very much alike. In fact, up until about the seventh week of development all babies look the same. After nine weeks, babies destined to be boys begin to make *testosterone,* the hormone that causes the male genitals to develop. If there's no testosterone, the baby will develop female genitals. In a way, you can think of his body as an "overgrown" version of your own. The chart below shows the male and female equivalent structures.

Female	Male
Clitoris	Penis
Glans of clitoris	Glans of penis
Shaft of clitoris	Shaft of penis
Crura of clitoris	Crura of penis
Vestibular bulb	Bulb of penis
Labia majora	Scrotum
Labia minora and clitoral bulb	Corpus spongiosum
Ovaries	Testicles
Peri-urethral glands	Prostate gland

Though the erect penis is sometimes called a "boner," there's not a bone to be found in it. And, despite how athletic it might seem, it has no muscles, either. Like the clitoris, the penis has two crura, a shaft and a head. The shaft is made up of a trio of cylinders composed of spongelike tissue that contains many blood vessels and nerves. They may not be obvious when the penis is soft but are more noticeable when the penis is erect. If you look at a flaccid penis as it hangs down in front of the scrotum, the side of the shaft facing you contains two of these cylinders, the *corpora cavernosa,* lying side by side and covered by a thick fibrous layer. As with the clitoris, the penis's corpora cavernosa end in two crura, or legs, that attach to the pubic bone.

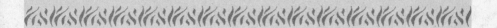

Circumcision

Whether for religious, cultural, or personal reasons, most boys in the United States these days are circumcised (the foreskin is removed) usually during the first few days after birth. If you are accustomed to seeing only circumcised penises, one that hasn't had the foreskin removed may look abnormal, but both work equally well during sex.

The foreskin produces an oily substance to lubricate the head of the penis. When this oil mixes with dead skin cells, it becomes a cheesy white substance called *smegma*. Smegma isn't dirty, and there's no truth to the myth that sex with an uncircumcised man increases your risks of cervical cancer or sexually transmitted infections. In fact, it may contain substances that fight bacteria and viruses, but if it isn't regularly removed through daily washing, it can accumulate and cause infections, odor, irritations, and pain in the penis.

If you lift the penis up against the abdomen and look at its underside, you'll see the third and smaller spongy cylinder, the *corpus spongiosum*. It becomes an obvious ridge on the underside of the penis when it is erect. The bottom of the corpus spongiosum forms the *bulb* of the penis. You can feel the bulb between the anus and the scrotum when the penis is erect. The top of the corpus spongiosum forms the mushroom-shaped *glans*—the soft, smooth head of the penis. If you look at the top of the head, you will notice a small slitlike opening leading to the urethra, a tube that runs through the middle of the corpora spongiosum to carry urine and semen out of the body. Unless he has had a circumcision, a layer of loose, elastic skin—hairless and usually several shades darker than the man himself—covers the penis, continuing over the glans as the foreskin, or *prepuce*.

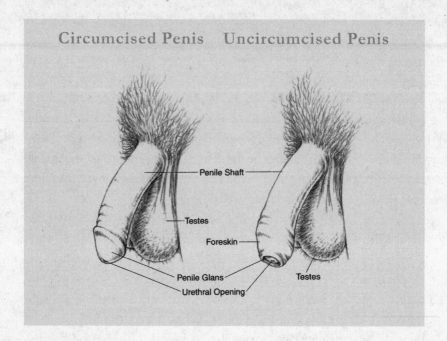

Circumcised Penis   Uncircumcised Penis

Penile Shaft

Testes

Foreskin

Penile Glans

Urethral Opening

Testes

Scrotum

The penis rests on top of the *scrotum,* a loose sac of skin and smooth muscle that's divided into two compartments, each containing one testicle. Darker in color than the rest of a man's skin, the scrotum is covered with fine hair as well as sweat- and oil-secreting glands. It may be loose and wrinkled or shiny. The muscle layer is responsible for pulling the scrotum up closer to the body when a man is exposed to cold temperatures or is frightened, or just about to ejaculate.

Testes

Also known as "balls," "nuts," "family jewels," and "sacks," the *testes* do bear some resemblance to your ovaries: They are egg-shaped, smooth, and measure about 2 inches across. You may notice that one testicle hangs lower in the scrotal pouch than the other. Most commonly the left testicle hangs lower, but in some men (most commonly left-handed people), the right one hangs lower. Like the ovaries, which make female hormones for

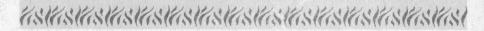

Testing the Testes

Becoming familiar with your partner's testes can save his life. While men should examine their testes on a regular basis for signs of testicular cancer, few of them do. Examining his testes for him can be a wonderful, sensual way to show that you care.

Gently grasp one testicle between your thumb and fingers. Slowly roll the testicle between your fingers and look for lumps, bumps, and areas that are tender, hard, or irregular in shape. Now repeat the same on the other side and compare the two testes. Any changes in the testes should be reported to a doctor. Testicular cancer occurs most commonly in men under the age of forty.

women, the testes make the major sex hormone for men, testosterone. They also produce millions of sperm daily, which are stored in a small area on the back of each testicle called the *epididymis*.

Some men like to have their testes fondled and gently sucked. But if you've ever had your ovaries squeezed during a pelvic exam, you know how uncomfortable it can be. The testes are just as sensitive to pressure, so they must be handled carefully. Squeeze too hard and you may cause a quick end to a romantic evening. Again, every man is different, and it is best to ask him whether he likes to have his testes handled.

Prostate Gland

The *prostate gland* is a small, firm organ, approximately the size and shape of a walnut, that sits at the bottom of the bladder. It produces a white fluid that helps sperm survive in the vagina. You can feel the prostate by placing your finger as far as you can in his rectum and running it down the front wall. Many men find stroking of the area surrounding, and including, the prostate to be highly pleasurable.

Prostate problems, including prostate enlargement and cancer, are common among older men, so if your partner is forty or older, encourage him to have a yearly prostate exam. A blood test called PSA (prostate-specific antigen) can help to detect prostate cancer early.

Sensitivity of the Penis

Like the clitoris, the penis is well innervated with nerves and very sensitive. Though the entire length of the penis is sensitive to touch, pressure, and temperature, the glans, or head, is more responsive than the shaft. And the rim of the head, called the *corona,* is the most sensitive of all. If you really want to drive your lover wild, look for the web of tissue on the back of the penis where the head meets the shaft, called the *frenulum.* Rubbing, massaging, and licking this area sends most men into orbit. Of course, all men are different, and some men may find that direct stimulation of the most sensitive parts of their penis is uncomfortable. It's always best to ask before you plunge in.

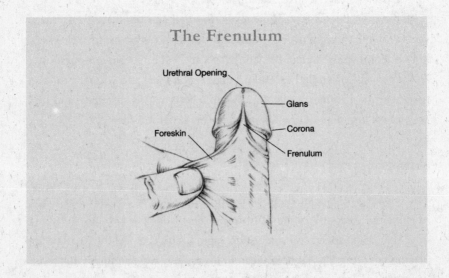

The Frenulum

Urethral Opening

Glans

Foreskin

Corona

Frenulum

Injury to the Penis

The skin covering the penis is elastic; it stretches, becoming taut and thin as the penis enlarges during erections. This tender skin may become scraped if, during prolonged, vigorous sex, the vagina becomes dry. These abrasions or friction burns can cause a tender scab to form on the shaft of the penis the day after sex. I have seen many women who have been accused of transmitting a sexually transmitted disease when their partners discovered such a scar. Use vaginal lubricants to prevent this injury, and avoid the headache—for you and your partner.

Erection

When a man is sexually aroused, the arteries in the penis dilate and blood comes rushing into his penis, filling the spaces in the three spongy cylinders. The blood flowing in creates pressure in the corpora cavernosa, which become longer and wider. As the pressure increases in the corpora, the veins that usually take blood away from the penis are pressed against the fibrous covering, so the blood that continues to rush into the penis can't leave. Thus the penis becomes larger and erect. The tough fibrous layer surrounding the corpora cavernosa becomes tense, making the penis rigid and hard.

During erection, most of the corpus spongiosum remains softer than the rest of the penis; however, the bulb becomes quite hard and sensitive. The head increases in size, becomes much darker in color, but remains somewhat soft. A rock-hard head probably wouldn't feel as good and could potentially damage the vagina and cervix.

Men do not have to be sexually aroused to experience an erection. Erections may occur when he is frightened, nervous, or when he has a full bladder. It's normal for men to have several erections during the dream phase of sleep, and they often wake up in the morning with a boner. Sometimes erections occur for no apparent reason. Just because he has a hard-on, it doesn't mean he is thinking about or ready for sex.

You may have noticed that sometimes during sex (oral, manual, or intercourse) your partner's penis becomes soft and then hard again. That doesn't mean he's not enjoying the encounter. It is normal for the penis to go through cycles of very firm to softer and firm again in some men. In fact it is not necessary for your man to get a hard-on at all to have fun. There are a lot of things you can do with a soft penis. You just need a little imagination.

Things to Do with a Soft Penis

Even when the penis is soft, most men, including impotent men, can experience pleasurable sensations and sometimes an orgasm. And a soft penis can provide a multitude of wonderful sensations for a woman. Try some of these:

- Lick and suck. When the penis is soft, it's much easier to get the whole thing in your mouth without gagging.

- Lubricate your hands and massage the shaft and head.

- Sit on top of him and stuff his penis into your vagina. Now slowly rotate your pelvis in small circles without lifting up. As you rotate, press your clitoris against his pubic bone.

- Squat over your partner (or have him squat over you), grab his penis at the base with your hand. Rub the head of the penis back and forth against your clitoris and vaginal opening.

- Have him lie flat with his legs straight. Place the penis up against his pubic bone or lower abdomen. Now straddle his pelvis and lower your vulva, spread your labia, and place your clitoris on top of the soft penis and rub back and forth. If he finds the full weight of your body too much, raise up a bit onto your knees for

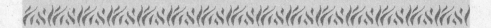

Fracture of the Penis

Even though the penis has no bone, it can be "broken." Fracture of the penis occurs when the penis is erect and most commonly during vigorous, athletic intercourse with the woman on top. The penis comes all of the way out and misses the opening on the way back in, causing it to ram the woman's pubic bone or other firm body part. A snapping or cracking sound is usually heard as the layer that surrounds the three spongy cylinders ruptures and blood is released underneath the skin of the penis, causing severe pain and swelling. *Fracture of the penis is considered a surgical emergency. The tear needs to be repaired immediately, so if this happens to your partner, rush him to the hospital.* Recovery is usually excellent, and men can return to normal sexual relations in a short period of time. Fortunately, this condition is rare.

support. Lean forward to give him kisses and massage his chest and arms.

Be creative and playful; enjoy the moment and don't make his erection a goal. Taking the pressure off him to have an erection may be his greatest turn-on.

Ejaculation

When your partner is at the peak of sexual arousal, he may orgasm and release seminal fluid in a process called *ejaculation*. Ejaculation begins with contraction of the muscles surrounding the tubes that transport sperm and semen. The sperm leave the epididymis and are propelled through the *vas deferens,* a long muscular tube that carries the sperm from the testicle to the urethra. As the vas deferens passes through the prostate gland, the

What's in Semen?

As you stimulate a sexually aroused man, you may notice a few drops of clear fluid seep from the tip of the penis. This is not semen. This fluid is released from small glands on the side of the urethra and helps sperm survive by lubricating the urethra and making it more alkaline. While this fluid doesn't contain sperm, sometimes sperm lurking in the urethra from a previous ejaculation are included in these early drops of fluid. That's why you need contraception throughout intercourse, not just at the time of ejaculation, to prevent an unintended pregnancy.

When a man actually ejaculates, he releases about a teaspoon of milky, whitish fluid called *semen,* which contains millions of sperm. Mostly, however, it consists of the fluid from the seminal vesicles and prostate gland, which contains vitamins, minerals, sugars, acids, bases, and salt. It has a distinctive but mild odor and is safe to swallow. The taste and scent of semen vary among men and in the same man at different times. Diet, smoking, alcohol, and exercise can change the taste of semen. It's not fattening, providing between 10 and 30 calories per teaspoon.

Keep in mind that semen can also carry bacteria and viruses, so practice safer sex if you are not sure of his health status. Also know that even though it's white, semen leaves a pale yellow stain when it dries that is sometimes difficult to remove.

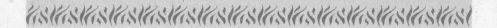

sperm pick up fluid from the gland and from two sacs called the *seminal vesicles.* The prostate gland contracts and propels the semen (fluid plus sperm) into the urethra. Then the pelvic floor muscles contract and send the semen flying out of the penis. The entire process (orgasm with ejaculation) lasts 5–10 seconds.

Some of my patients have voiced concern because their partners don't always ejaculate. I tell them not to worry; men don't always have to ejaculate in every sexual coupling. Some men can even have an orgasm without ejaculation. In fact, some consider control over their ejaculations to be an advantage in lovemaking, allowing them to make love for longer periods of time and more frequently. Tantric and Taoist philosophies suggest that ejaculatory control helps men to increase their sexual energy, create more powerful orgasms, and experience a greater spiritual, loving connection to their partner.

The bottom line is that it doesn't mean that you have failed as a sex partner or that he doesn't care for you if he doesn't "come." If your man is happy, don't make an issue of it. But if it's causing a problem in the relationship, consider seeing a sex therapist.

The Issue of Size

The male obsession with penis size begins early. To make my point, I will share the conversation I overheard between my three sons as they stepped out of the shower.

"Your penis is short. Mine is much bigger than yours," said my six-year-old to his nine-year-old brother.

"Is not!" he exclaimed.

My four-year-old, aware of his disadvantage, ran to the next room and returned with a small magnifying glass from a toy science kit. He placed it directly in front of his penis and exclaimed, "Look! Mine is the biggest of all!"

Many boys grow up, as my sons did, comparing themselves to one another. By the time they are men, they've learned to believe that a large penis makes them more masculine, better lovers, and more desirable; so they're almost always curious to see how they measure up.

The female obsession with penis size begins later, but we do indeed obsess. From the time we become sexually active, many of us believe that "bigger is better" and that a big penis will make us have multiple glorious orgasms. The truth is size doesn't matter. Remember the vagina is a potential space that can stretch, grasp, and envelope almost any size penis. Even if his penis is small, if he knows how to move it, he can hit all of your most sensitive spots and give you tremendous pleasure. He can be as big as a mule but, without any technique, will leave you cold. As they say, "It's not what you've got but what you do with it."

The size of the average penis has been greatly exaggerated with the help of romance novels and pornographic movies. The average penis measures between 2 and 4 inches long when it's soft. It can appear even shorter if a man is overweight (the surrounding fat can obscure the true length of the penis), and if he's cold, anxious, or nervous, you may notice a temporary "shrinkage" of his organ.

Looking at the size of a soft penis doesn't give you the complete picture because the soft size isn't necessarily proportional to the erect size. A small penis will grow proportionately more than a large one when hard. For example, a man with a penis that's 3 inches long when it's soft can produce a penis of 6 inches or more when hard. A man with a 5-inch penis when soft may grow less when hard, so both men may end up the same size when erect.

When it's erect, the typical penis measures between 4 and 6 inches long and 4–5 inches around, and they can vary in shape. Some have big heads and small shafts; some have big shafts and small heads; and some are the same all the way down. When hard, some of them stick straight out from the body like a flagpole; some angle up toward the belly; and a few point down toward the ground even when erect. They may be slightly curved to the left or the right, up or down. It doesn't matter. They all work when placed in the vagina, a very accommodating organ.

If his penis is markedly curved, however, he may have Peyronie's disease. Doctors don't know what causes this, though we think it may result from repeated trauma to the penis, which causes scars to form and the penis to curve. (No, chronic masturbation will not cause Peyronie's disease.) If a man has it, erection and intercourse may be painful, but fortunately the disease can be surgically corrected.

What to Do with What He's Got

Whether he's large or small, curved or straight, he can be a great lover if he—and you—know how to make the most of his endowments. Remember that women come in different shapes and sizes, too. Your vagina may be long and narrow or wide and spacious—and the nature of that cavity may differ from adolescence to motherhood to menopause. Following are the recommendations that I give my patients when they voice concern about the size of their partner's penis.

Small Penis

The woman who's with a man who has a relatively small penis usually complains that she doesn't feel much pressure deep within the vagina during sex. The penis may even "fall out." My advice is to choose positions where the depth of penetration can be the greatest. If you're on the bottom, pull your knees all the way up against your chest and/or place a pillow under your buttocks. Also, use your pelvic floor muscles to grip the penis as the two of you move. You can sit on his penis and straddle his hips as he lies flat. Or he can enter you from the rear while you are on hands and knees.

Big Penis

Despite the "bigger is better" myth, some women complain that sex with a well-endowed man is uncomfortable. If this is your situation, make sure that you are relaxed and engage in lots of foreplay before intercourse because as you become more excited, the vagina becomes longer and wider. Foreplay will also generate more lubrication, which will facilitate a smoother entrance. Alternately, use a water-soluble lubricant inside the vagina as well as on the surface of the penis. Go slowly.

Choose positions in which the depth of penetration is shallower. For example, lie on the top or bottom with your legs straight and use your inner thigh muscles to stimulate the penis. Your inner thighs and labia will add "length" to your vagina. Getting on top will give you the most control of the depth of penetration.

Part II

Sensational
Sex

Chapter 4

Sensational, Sensual, Satisfying Sex

Sex is a banquet, a smorgasbord of unlimited pleasures to choose from.

—Miriam Biddleman, sex therapist

What Is Sex?

Ask one hundred people to define *sex* and most will define it as "intercourse," "coitus," or some sort of joining of the genitals. For most people, all other intimate activities fall into the category of foreplay, meaning they are the opening acts for the main sexual event—appetizers before the main course, if you will. While some people debate whether or not oral sex or masturbation qualifies as sex, I define sex broadly to include a generous number of pleasurable, sensual activities.

When you get right down to it, any intimate physical contact designed to give erotic pleasure is sex. Amorous touching is sex. Sensual kissing is sex. Tasting your partner's intimate juices is sex. So if any of my patients begin to talk about sex only as it relates to the genitals, I remind them that any sensual activity is as important as the next and that many of these sexy pleasures need not end with intercourse. Stroking the body of your lover can be just as sensuous and gratifying as intercourse, if not more so. Remember when you were a teenager how thrilling it was to spend an evening kissing on the sofa or in the backseat of a car? Who says that you can't enjoy that kind of pleasure now? Even if your teenage years are long past, an innocent necking session can be a wonderful way to bring excitement back into your love life. There are endless ways to share erotic pleasures with your partner. The more of these techniques (and variations) you know about, practice, and master, the more fantastic a sex life you can expect to have.

That's why I've included a step-by-step guide to each sexual technique and variation. It's true that good sex should not be mechanical or technical, but to be a great lover—and to receive the best possible pleasure from your lovemaking—you need to be aware of some basic lovemaking skills. If you want to play the flute, you must learn where to put your fingers and how to blow on the hole. In the beginning you may feel a little awkward, but with a little instruction and practice, you can become a virtuoso. It's the same with sex.

In this section, I describe sexual intimacies as "delicacies," and intercourse is but one of the many delights. With this menu, there are no rules. You can have desert before the appetizer and the after-dinner mints before the entrée. Or start with the main course, then try a little dessert, then go back to the main course and end with the appetizer. It can be a banquet or a barbecue. It's up to you to decide. If it's true that "variety is the spice of life," you're sure to have a very tantalizing, delicious sex life.

Playing by the "Rules"

Often it's "the rules"— our notions about what one should or should not do in bed—that keep us from fully enjoying our sexuality. I try to get my patients to let go of that kind of sexually limited thinking, but there are a couple of rules that I ask them to honor always.

Rule Number One: Always communicate

Being able to express yourself with your partner is vital to a good sexual relationship. For example, when you're making love, let him know when he touches the right spot in the right way. That doesn't mean you have to have a long conversation about it; you can moan, sigh, or whisper his name. He'll probably get the message and appreciate the applause. Of course, if you're moaning with pain rather than pleasure, he needs to know that. And whatever you do, don't fake it. If he thinks he's pleasing you, he'll keep doing what he's doing. Likewise, you should also find out whether or not your moves are pleasing to your partner. That means you two have to talk about your sexual relationship—in bed and out.

Sex therapist Miriam Biddleman recommends this simple exercise for learning more about your sexual desires and those of your partner. First, each of you should make a list of what turns you on—the things you already enjoy doing together as well as things you'd like to try. Then make a similar list of what you *think* turns your partner on. Have fun reading the lists to each other and make mental notes for the next time you are intimate. You may find yourself pleasantly surprised—and excited—by your partner's unspoken desires.

Every woman's experience of sex is different. Sometimes sex is a magical, spiritual, out-of-body experience; at other times pleasure is focused in your physical feelings. Your lovemaking experience may change from day to day, year to year, or partner to partner, but it should always be a mutually enjoyable activity defined by the two people involved. I emphasize the word *mutual*, which brings us to rule number two:

Rule Number Two: Never allow yourself to be pressured into any activity that makes you uncomfortable, no matter what your partner may want

Yes, you may be a little nervous or awkward as you experiment and try new things, but whatever you do, remember that *you* are in charge of what you do sexually. There is no right or wrong way to have sex, and no one has the right to tell you how, when, where, or with whom to have sex. If it doesn't feel right, don't do it.

Talking to Your Partner About Sex

The key to fantastic sex is communication with your partner. That may sound easy, but most couples don't talk about sex. This is as true for couples who have been together for twenty years as for those who have just recently met. Most of us were raised in environments where sex was such a taboo subject that it continues to be taboo to talk about it—even if we're actually doing it! You may think it's embarrassing, or you may worry about what your partner will think of you or whether he will be hurt and feel that you are complaining. Taking the time to let your partner know what really turns you on and taking the time to learn what turns him on will help you achieve the sex life of your dreams.

Before trying to communicate your sexual needs and desires to your partner, it is vital that you take personal inventory of your sexual self. Do you like sex? Do you like sex with your partner? Do you know what gives you pleasure and what doesn't? Are you aware of your erogenous zones—not the ones highlighted in books on sex, but yours? It's really important to tell yourself the truth; there are no wrong answers here. But if you answered "no" to any of these questions, then it's time for you to begin to explore your body and discover what turns you on. You can begin to do this on your own at first. When you and your lover are receptive and open, then you can engage in exploration together.

Once you feel comfortable having a meaningful discussion with your partner about sex, be prudent about the circumstances under which you will be having your conversations. Pick a time when you're both relaxed and not under pressure. Don't have the conversation just after one of you has just walked in the door after work and is tired. If you are uneasy or irritable, pick another time. Never have important conversations in the car. And certainly don't have a dialogue about sex right before, during, or after sex—times when you are most likely to have charged emotions and feelings. Sex is best discussed outside the sexual environment.

And remember that talking with your partner isn't a gripe session; you're trying to get to some solutions for making your lovemaking more

Talking Points

Try these tips for breaking the ice about the subject of sex.

❧ Read a sex book together. Linger on the chapters that describe the techniques that you particularly enjoy. Say something like, "I just love it when you do that to me."

❧ Rent an erotic video and discuss the activities that entice you or pique your interest. Tell him, "I'd love to try that."

❧ Share your fantasies with each other. Describe in intimate detail activities that you find particularly pleasurable or would like to try.

❧ If he did something in bed that you particularly liked, let him know immediately after sex: "When you touched me that way it really drove me wild."

satisfying. Stress the positives and avoid complaints. Sex conversations should not be about who is doing something right or wrong. If you put your partner on the defensive, the dialogue is over.

Sometimes we expect our men to know everything about sex and depend on them to instinctively know what turns us on. Unless you take the time to share with your partner your likes, desires, fantasies, and all of your feelings about sex, you are cheating yourself out of a potentially extraordinary sexual relationship.

Sex is mutual. Like sex itself, your conversation should be between two people who would like to get closer, make sex better, and have a more meaningful and passionate sexual experience. If one of you is unwilling to work to make sex better, then your problem isn't sex. It's your relationship.

In my practice, I have seen many women who suffer in silence. This silence sometimes leads not only to unsatisfying sex but also to injuries. If your partner is doing something that you find uncomfortable, let him know. Don't say things like "I hate the way you do that" or "You're doing it all wrong." Gently, but firmly, move his hand or body to an area that you find more pleasurable. Put your hand on top of his and gently, lovingly change the location, direction, pressure, or tempo of his movements. When he gets it just right, moan your deepest moan or whisper in his ear letting him know how much pleasure he is giving you.

Setting the Scene

You can have great sex spontaneously on a kitchen table covered with yesterday's leftovers, but some of the most mind-blowing sexual experiences involve a bit of planning. How you prepare for a romantic encounter with your lover reflects who you are, and taking time to prepare a special experience for your partner lets him or her know that you care. Your plans don't have to be exotic, expensive, time consuming, or over the top; it's just important that you do something that shows your partner that your feelings are genuine and strong. The idea is to set a mood for pleasuring each other. When you create the right ambiance, your largest sex organ—the brain—and all of your senses are stimulated, and sex becomes a total body experience.

Creating a romantic retreat—even in your own bedroom—can be a wonderful way to introduce sex to a new relationship or to spice up a love affair that has seen better days. You're preparing a special place that encourages you to tune out the outside world so you're free to focus totally on the experience of lovemaking. Turn off the phone and your beeper, lock the door, ask Grandma to take the kids for the evening. Then get creative. As you prepare the space for lovemaking, remember that you want to stimulate more than just the genitals. If you first find romantic and sexy ways to stroke and stimulate each of the five senses, you'll soon find that you and your partner will be carried away in waves of passion.

Sight

If you use your imagination and are creative, you'll find dozens of ways to stimulate your partner's sense of sight. Dim lighting has always been associated with romance, so keep the lighting soft and indirect. Use a dimmer switch on your lights, if you have one, or put low-wattage bulbs in your lamps. If you want to create a "hot" mood, use red lightbulbs. And everyone looks more beautiful in candlelight, so position candles around the room. (But be aware of fire hazards.)

Everyone knows that flowers thrill most women, but we don't often think of them as pleasing men as well. A large bouquet near your love nest will please both of you with its beauty and fragrance. Sprinkle fresh red rose petals over the bed or, better yet, strew them between the sheets for a surprise.

For drama, turn your bed into a temple by draping sensuous fabrics across the bed or from the ceiling over the bed. For Oriental exoticism, arrange a brilliantly colored silk kimono across the bed and top it with a string of white pearls. Or bring a variety of large plants into the bedroom to create a wild "jungle" or dense rainforest—a Garden of Eden just for the two of you.

Here's a surprising finding: A study has shown that the testosterone levels and the level of arousal increased in some men when they viewed pictures of their favorite sports team. In fact, men were almost as aroused as if they'd viewed erotic photos. So if he loves baseball, place a large bat, a baseball, and a picture of his favorite team on or near the bed.

Of course, what you wear can also be a turn-on, but you don't have to dress like a Playboy centerfold to make him drool. Showing up occasionally wearing nothing but a thong can be a part of your repertoire, but generally you'd do well to wear something made from a soft fabric—a garment that is flattering but leaves a lot to the imagination.

Smell

Think of how you react to the smell of fresh-baked bread, a meal home-cooked by your mother, a vase of fresh roses, your lover's cologne. Some say that scent is second only to touch in its power to arouse feelings in people. So infuse your love nest with wonderful fragrances to arouse passionate feelings in your beloved. Ylang-ylang, jasmine, Sandalwood, rose, patchouli, cedarwood, lavender, or clary sage are some specific scents have been shown to excite the senses and act as sexual stimulants in the brain. Place sachets or candles containing these fragrances around the room. Or put these essential oils in an infuser over your lightbulbs; the heat will release the fragrance into the air.

Oddly enough, studies also have shown that men are turned on by the scent of cinnamon buns, strawberries, cola, and vanilla. Bake a batch of fresh cinnamon buns and let their warm fragrance be the first thing he smells when he walks in the door. I've heard of women who dab a little vanilla extract at pulse points (and other places) the way they would perfume. Of course, each person's fragrance preferences are different. If it's fresh-baked bread he loves, get your hands on some dough. He adores your perfume? Spray some on the pillows and sheets.

Sound

Music can have a marked effect on our moods. Soft music can be quite romantic; something with a steady, pulsing rhythm can inspire powerful, passionate lovemaking. You might want to find music that you can dance to—for him or with him. Middle-Eastern belly-dancing music, African rhythms, or certain reggae numbers can get your hips moving in ways that will delight your partner. Just the right sexy, sax-y jazz number can get the two of you moving in perfect synch. Choose music that you both find pleasant, nondistracting, and sensual—music you *both* like. The wrong tune can be distracting and a turn-off.

These days you can also find "environmental" sounds—recordings of rivers or waves splashing against the beach—that can add to the ambiance you want to create for your love lair and help drown out distracting noises. Then, too, sometimes silence, interrupted only by deep breathing and sighs of pleasure, is the best sound imaginable.

Touch

Touch is the strongest of all senses during sex; in fact the nerve endings in your skin are more sensitive to touch when you're aroused. Above all, you'll want to touch and be touched by your partner. We'll talk more about touch when we get to the sexual delicacies. Just make sure that you choose a comfortable place for lovemaking. Sex on the beach can be thrilling—unless you're suffering abrasions from the sand. If you think you'll end up in the bed, make sure the sheets are fresh and clean, smooth and soft.

Satin is especially sensuous, but a good-quality, high-thread-count cotton can be just as nice. Look for the same smooth comfort in the clothing you wear to bed as well as in the things you use for erotic play. Inspect anything you plan to use as a sex toy to make sure there are no sharp edges or parts that will chafe or irritate you or your partner. For different and erotic sensations, stroke your lover's bare skin with feathers, silk, leather, or fur.

Taste

Perhaps the most delicious thing you can bring to your lovemaking session is yourself and your partner. If you're in love, the very taste of your partner's lips is arousing; your own natural juices are probably tantalizing to him or her as well. But if you want to add flavor, feed each other chocolates, berries, or savory morsels. Drizzle each other with honey, syrup, or whipped cream that can be licked and kissed away. Don't put these inside the vagina, however; they can be difficult to remove and may cause infections.

When and Where

It's not necessary to have a bed to have intercourse. In fact, some of your most fun and exciting sex will occur outside the bedroom. Where exactly? You are only limited by your imagination. My patients have given me all sorts of ideas about exciting places to have sex. Try some of these:

In Water A great place to have intercourse is in a swimming pool, ocean, hot tub, Jacuzzi, or bathtub. The water gives you a sense of weightlessness and increases the intensity of your lovemaking. I often recommend a romp in the bathtub for a woman's first act of intercourse, since the warm water is relaxing and soothing. It is also a natural lubricant, making insertion of the penis easier.

Under Water Take a shower together. Try using the showerhead to stimulate your clitoris while he enters your vagina from the rear.

On Water Get together on the deck of a sailboat. Don't forget the sunscreen.

In the Car Many women have fantasies of making love in a parked car—probably left over from the naughty excitement of high school encounters. And today's cars have seats that will recline all the way back, making it quite comfortable even for those of us who are no longer teenagers. If you can afford a limo, you're golden!

Anywhere Else You're limited only by how daring you are—and how athletic.

- On the stairs: Better going up than down.
- In an elevator: A quickie perhaps?
- In the woods: What a way to connect with nature!
- On the bathroom floor: Be careful that you don't slip.

Sex During Your Period

There is no reason why a woman who craves sex during her menses should deny herself sexual gratification. And here's a good reason to go ahead and do it: Sex and orgasm have been shown to be instant cures for menstrual cramps and menstrual migraines. Even if you don't have intercourse, don't hesitate to curl up with your beloved. Touch and massage increase the release of pain-relieving endorphins from the brain.

Oral sex is also okay during your period. Some men like the taste of iron in the menstrual blood. Just make sure he doesn't blow air into your vagina. Air may be forced into your bloodstream, travel to your lungs, and affect your heart (an air embolus).

Many women shy from intercourse during their period because it is "messy." A diaphragm or cervical cap will decrease the amount of blood that escapes during sex. Place a towel under your bottom to protect your sheets.

You may find that positions that cause very deep penetration are somewhat uncomfortable. The pelvic organs become slightly swollen during your period and may be more sensitive in some women.

Despite popular wisdom, it is possible to get pregnant during your period. If your menstrual cycles are short (21–25 days) or your periods are long (more than 7 days), you may ovulate before you stop bleeding, and sperm can live up to 5 days in the vagina. And if your periods are irregular, it may be difficult to predict exactly when you will ovulate. So make sure you have contraception if you are not ready for an unplanned pregnancy. Foams, creams, and gels placed in the vagina will be less effective due to the blood flow and should not be used alone.

During your period the opening to the cervix and uterus is more accessible. Harmful sexually transmitted bacteria have easier access to your uterus, increasing your risks of a serious pelvic infection. Human immunodeficiency virus is also more easily transmitted during your period. If you are not sure about his infection status, use a condom.

Chapter 5

Increasing Your Pleasure: In Search of the Big "O"

I was engaged, married (for six years), divorced, single, and engaged again before I experienced the big "O"! Furthermore I didn't know what was happening and I was scared and cried. I'll never forget it—Nags Head, North Carolina, Memorial Day 1968!

—Anonymous

It wasn't long ago when women who had orgasms were considered abnormal. Before long, a woman was considered abnormal if she didn't have them. And, of course, you had to be able to have the *right* kind of orgasm. First you needed to have a vaginal orgasm to be normal, then simultaneous orgasms were the goal. Soon multiple orgasms took the limelight only to be replaced by extended, massive, all-night orgasms. And doctors are close to perfecting remote-controlled medical implants that can be placed in your spine and will allow you to give yourself an orgasm whenever you want one.

With all the hype about orgasms, the focus on the emotional and spiritual connection between two people went out the window. Achieving an orgasm or more orgasms has become the goal of sex play for many couples. And many women find the pressure to perform to be distracting and stressful—the exact opposite of how they need to feel in order to come to that kind of climax. What should be an intensely pleasurable experience becomes work.

But sex is about pleasure, and pleasure takes many forms. There are many perfectly satisfied women who have fulfilling sex lives without orgasm. For them, orgasm may not be the main source of sexual satisfaction. The intimacy, physical closeness, caring, and love that you share with your partner can be fulfilling in its own right. Every woman must decide for herself what her own needs and desires are.

What Is an Orgasm?

Orgasm, also known as "climax" or "coming," is described by Masters and Johnson as the point in the female response cycle when accumulated sexual tension is released. Physically, orgasm consists of a series of rhythmic contractions of the uterus, lower vagina, and pelvic floor muscles. Though orgasm is always described as highly pleasurable, it may be experienced differently by different women. Some women have orgasms but don't realize it because they are expecting "bombs to go off" like they do in the romance novels or movies. For some women, the sensations are localized in the pelvis. Others may experience mental imagery, auras, or brief loss of consciousness. Each orgasmic experience, though, ends with sexual satisfaction and relaxation.

Orgasmic Truths

Between 10 and 12 percent of women in America have never experienced an orgasm. And the majority of women who do have them don't achieve orgasm during vaginal intercourse alone. Penis-in-vagina intercourse is just not a very effective way of achieving orgasm for most women. For most women, stimulation of the clitoris is necessary to achieve orgasm. Some find stimulation of the G-spot or other areas of the vagina to hold the trigger to orgasm. Still others can orgasm through stimulation of the nipples, vulva, other nongenital erogenous zones or through fantasy.

Many women find orgasm through masturbation to be more intense than orgasm through intercourse, and most of us find it easiest to orgasm during manual stimulation or oral sex. There is no one right way to achieve orgasm. I see women weekly who fear that something is wrong with them or that they are missing something if they only orgasm through manual stimulation or oral sex. Physically, an orgasm is an orgasm is an orgasm. It is the same whether it is in response to oral sex, manual stimulation, intercourse, or fantasy. And an orgasm achieved through intercourse is no more valid or special than one achieved through clitoral stimulation.

The majority of women who are capable of achieving orgasm through intercourse are not orgasmic every time. And the intensity of orgasm can vary from one episode to the other. Sometimes it may be strong and long, and other times it may be barely perceptible.

Making simultaneous orgasms a goal can ruin your enjoyment of the sexual experience. You may become so preoccupied with the task that pleasure eludes you. Your only goal should be to let go and enjoy giving and receiving pleasure from your partner.

Female Ejaculation

Though the concept remains somewhat controversial, and most Western-trained physicians don't believe that it happens, there is evidence that some women do, in fact, "ejaculate" a fluid at the time of orgasm.

Hundreds of years ago, Aristotle concluded that women release a fluid during orgasm. Then, in 1950, Dr. Ernest Grafenberg found that stimulation of the front wall of the vagina—the G spot— could trigger orgasm and the expulsion of a thin fluid anywhere from a few drops to more than a cup. Studies support his finding and indicate that from 10–40 percent of women release fluid from the urethra during orgasm.

Most researchers think the fluid comes from the system of glands and ducts that surrounds the urethra and develops from the same tissue as the prostate gland in the male. And while some studies have shown the fluid to be indistinguishable from urine, others have shown it to be distinct and to contain an enzyme that is typically found only in the prostatic component of male urine.

Ejaculation shouldn't become something you strive for during sex; if it happens, it happens. But if you have been embarrassed by what you have assumed was incontinence of urine when you have sex, don't worry. You could be one of those women who ejaculates.

The Importance of Masturbation

Anna is a seventy-three-year-old woman who came to my office for a routine yearly exam. "Before I die, I want to see what it feels like to have an orgasm," she said. Though she considered her past sex life to have been fulfilling, she had never had an orgasm. She was not sexually active and had not been for more than thirteen years. She had never masturbated.

We started with a lesson in sexual anatomy. With the use of a mirror, she was instructed to examine her vulva, clitoris, and vaginal opening. It was the first time that she had looked, and she was thrilled by the sight of her genitals. She was not taking estrogen and had thinning and dryness of her vulva and vagina. I prescribed daily massages of her vulva with estrogen cream and oral hormone replacement therapy (estrogen and progesterone). Through the Internet, she ordered Betty Dodson's video *Celebrating Orgasm,* an electric vibrator, two water-based lubricants, and an erotic video.

After several weeks of estrogen therapy, it was time to advance to the next step in her "journey of self discovery." I told her how to use the lubricant to stroke, massage, and discover the areas of her sexual anatomy that brought her the most pleasure. She was a little reluctant to self-stimulate because of her upbringing, but she was very motivated to achieve orgasm. I instructed her to watch the two videos, self-stimulate, and use the vibrator.

Two weeks passed before I heard from Anna. She had experienced several "glorious" orgasms. But she was "mad as hell" with her ex-husband who "never told her what she was missing."

Self-Pleasuring

The first step in increasing your pleasure during sex and learning how to achieve orgasm is to learn how to self-pleasure. Learning what turns you on, what gives you pleasure, and where your trigger points are will make it easier for you to have enjoyable and satisfying sex, alone or with your partner.

Plan your self-pleasuring for a time when you can be completely alone, without interruptions or distractions. Take the phone off the hook and don't answer the door. Make yourself comfortable by using pillows and blankets. Using a water-based lubricant or an unscented oil, begin with your mons and labia majora. Stroke and massage, being aware of the sensations that loving your genitals brings. Slide your fingers along your labia minora. Slide along the sides of your clitoris, along the body and glans.

Begin with a light feathery touch and gradually increase the pressure as you move your hands. Try different speeds. Vary the direction of your strokes from up and down to side-to-side to circular motions. Concentrate only on the pleasurable sensations that you feel. If you don't feel pleasurable sensations, don't be discouraged. It sometimes takes several self-pleasuring sessions before you begin to relax and receive the wonderful sensations that your body is capable of producing.

There are several ways to increase your arousal, muscle tension, and enjoyment during self-pleasuring. Experiment and find what works best for you.

- Use fantasy to increase your arousal and help you to concentrate on erotic sensations.

- An erotic woman-sensitive video or erotic literature may help to focus your thoughts on pleasure.

- Contract and release your pelvic floor muscles during self-stimulation to increase blood flow and arousal. It may also make orgasm easier and more intense.

- Add stimulation of your breasts and nipples.

- Vary your breathing. Some women find that panting rapidly increases their arousal.

- Move your pelvis. Rotating your hips during self-pleasuring may loosen you up and help you hit just the right spots to bring you intense pleasure.

The most important thing to remember in self-pleasuring is that orgasm is not the goal. Relax and take your time. Some men, and a few women, can orgasm after only a couple of minutes of stimulation, while some women may take an hour or more. Self-pleasuring is one exercise that you can practice and practice without having to worry about a partner's pleasure or his timetable. Each time you do it, you increase your pleasure and knowledge of what turns you on. Enjoy the journey of self-discovery, and in time orgasm will follow.

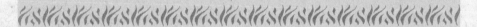

Did You Know:
Masturbation Facts

❧ Masturbation is a natural healthy part of sexual behavior for people of all ages.

❧ Masturbation was once thought to cause insanity, hair loss, acne, heart disease, seizure, idiocy, blindness, warts, memory loss, physical weakness, and hairy palms.

❧ Married people are more likely to masturbate than people living alone (NHSLS survey), so if you discover that he occasionally pleasures himself, don't take it as a personal rejection.

❧ Masturbation increases blood flow to your genitals and makes orgasms easier to achieve.

Other Ways to Self-Stimulate

Vibrator

Sex therapists recommend using a vibrator if you have been unable to achieve orgasm through manual self-stimulation. Vibrators can also add a new dimension to your sex life. A vibrator may be especially helpful for postmenopausal women who may need the intense stimulation that a vibrator provides to reach orgasm.

Pillow Talk

Place a firm pillow between your legs. Thrust or grind your pelvis and vulva against the pillow. If you don't have a pillow, a folded towel works as well.

Water Games

Warm water can be soothing and stimulating. Lie in the bathtub and position your pelvis so that a gentle flow of water is directed between your legs and against your vulva. You may need to place your legs and feet against the wall to get into the right position. As you become more aroused, you might want to increase the force of the flow of water against your vulva and clitoris. The warmth of the water will also increase the blood flow to your genitals and increase your arousal.

A handheld showerhead can be used to direct warm water against your vulva. Start with a light spray of water. As you become more aroused you may increase the amount of water, or if there is a massage option you can change the intensity of the water spray. Do not shoot water directly into your vagina; it can increase your risks of vaginal and pelvic infections.

Maneuver your vulva so that it is in the direct path of a water jet in a Jacuzzi or hot tub. The water is under a lot of pressure, so you don't want to get too close to the jets.

Crossing Your Legs

While sitting in a chair, cross your legs tightly at your knees. Rhythmically contract and relax your inner thigh muscles. Your clitoris will be trapped and squeezed by your thigh muscles. You can practice this method anytime, anywhere, and no one will be the wiser.

Tips to Increase Orgasm During Intercourse

Intercourse can be intensely pleasurable without orgasm, but if you'd like to increase your pleasure and the possibility that you will achieve orgasm during intercourse, try some of the following suggestions.

Masturbate in Front of Your Partner

Some women find it easy to orgasm during masturbation but less so during intercourse. Once you have learned to pleasure yourself, share this information with your partner. Showing your partner where your trigger points are and exactly what turns you on will make sex more pleasurable for both of you.

Clitoral Stimulation

You or your partner can stimulate your clitoris during intercourse. Rear entry and woman-on-top positions give you both easier access to your clitoris. For a change of pace, either of you can use a vibrator to stimulate your clitoris during intercourse.

Positions

Choose positions for intercourse that will increase stimulation of your most sensitive spots.

Woman-on-top

Gives you the most control during intercourse. You can direct the penis against your clitoris, G-spot, or any other area that gives you the most pleasure. You can control the depth of penetration, pressure, and tempo of intercourse.

Coital alignment technique (CAT)

Takes a little practice to get right but is worth the effort. Begin with the typical missionary position. After he has inserted his penis, he moves his pelvis forward so that his pelvis "overrides" yours. In this position, the base of his penis is pushed up against your clitoris. The pelvic movement is not the typical "in and out" thrusting but more of a rocking motion. You lead the upward stroke and he leads the downward stroke. His penis is in contact with your clitoris at all times.

Rear-entry

Increases stimulation of your G-spot.

Plan Sex

Planning sex can get your juices flowing before an encounter. You have all day—or all week—to think about how great it's going to be.

Fantasies

Share fantasies, erotic stories, books, and videos to increase your arousal. Fantasies help keep your mind focused on erotic stimulation and decrease distracting thoughts.

Connect with Your Partner

Spend time talking, hugging, and touching before intercourse. Most women need lots of foreplay before they can feel secure, safe, loved, relaxed, and sexually aroused enough to reach orgasm.

Live in the Moment

Concentrate totally on the sensations that you are experiencing during sex. Often we drift off to worries about whether we're pleasing our partner or whether we'll have an orgasm. It's okay to be "selfish" and concentrate on what you're feeling. The more you focus on the pleasurable sensations you are feeling, rather than what you think you should be feeling, the more likely you are to orgasm.

Kegel Exercises

Contract your pelvic floor muscles while having intercourse to increase blood flow and arousal. See Chapter 13 for details on how to practice Kegels.

Breathe

Learning how to breathe can add a new dimension to your lovemaking. Take a slow, deep breath, allowing your abdomen to expand and your lungs to fill completely. Now slowly release the breath. Allow yourself to make sounds as you exhale. Notice how your body begins to relax. Repeat the deep-breathing exercises but now increase the speed of your breathing. Studies have shown that rapid deep breathing during sex increases your sexual arousal and enjoyment.

Chapter 6
Delicacy #1: Kissing

Is there anything more sensual than a kiss? There are many different types of kisses, and each kiss can have a different meaning. A deep kiss signals the depth of your desire; even a soft brush of your lips can convey passion. There is no right or wrong way to do it, but every person has his or her likes and dislikes when it comes to kissing. The kind of kisses that turned your last lover to mush may not turn your current love on at all. Learning a variety of kissing techniques will make it easy for you to be a fantastic kisser with any partner. This section will help you expand your smooching skills—and help your partner do the same. Don't skip this section, thinking that you learned all you need to know about kissing in high school. Even if you're a perfectly good kisser, you can benefit from a refresher on an oft-neglected art.

Many women I know believe that a person's prowess as a kisser is a good indication of what kind of lover he or she is likely to be. They think that if a man doesn't know how to use his lips, he can't possibly have mastery over his other body parts. But before you turn a potentially lovely lover away because of his or her poor kisses, remember that, like anything else, kissing can be learned.

Most women love to kiss. That's usually the first intimate physical contact we have with a partner, and throughout our lives it continues to be a key part of lovemaking. Some women view kissing as more erotic and intimate than intercourse, in part because kissing conveys feelings of love and commitment in a way that intercourse alone does not. For others, kissing is only a step along the route to intercourse. Either way, it's true that kissing can be a real turn-on: It causes the release of *endorphins,* chemicals that make us feel good. And because it is both physically and emotionally stimulating—involving all of our senses at once—it may be the most potent aphrodisiac that a couple has at their disposal. In fact, kissing can be so sexually intense that a few women can orgasm from kissing alone. Unfortunately, the most common complaint among women regarding kissing is that they don't get enough of it. It is often the first intimate physical activity to be lost in short-term relationships that are suffering or long-term ones that have simply lost their spark.

Here are some of the ways to keep kissing a vital part of your sex life. Kissing can be innocent and flirtatious or a precursor to something more intimate.

Kissing and Your Senses

You breathe deeply and release a sigh, pulling away slightly, to look into your lover's eyes. You touch his face, running a finger along the edge of soft lips that you have just tasted. Then with pleasure you lean toward him, catching the scent of his natural pheromones, and begin covering him with soft, quiet kisses again.

When you are completely involved in kissing, it can encompass all your senses. The more aware you are of what pleases the senses, the better the experience will be for you and your partner.

Taste

Be conscious of how you're "flavoring" your kisses. Smoking, drinking alcohol, or eating spicy food, garlic, or onions prior to kissing can leave a disagreeable taste in your mouth that can turn off your partner. Drink plenty of water to keep your mouth fresh. If all else fails, suck on a mint or other sweet treat before you pucker up.

Smell

Some of the same foods, drinks, and habits that leave a bad taste in your mouth can also cause unpleasant odors—a sure turnoff. You know that poor dental hygiene and cavities can cause stay-away-from-me breath. But did you know that your breath may be particularly offensive if you are following a high-protein, low-carbohydrate diet? The first step to ending mouth odor is to thoroughly and frequently brush and floss your teeth and tongue. Dehydration causes stale mouth odor, so drink plenty of water. Sucking lemon drops will increase the saliva in your mouth and decrease mouth odor. Chewing parsley and sucking sugar-free mints can help cover offensive odors temporarily. If the problem persists, make sure to see your dentist.

Sight

Most women like to keep their eyes closed while kissing. However, watching your partner can add to the intimate, romantic nature of kissing. You may want to pull away from the kiss periodically to take an intimate, close-up gaze at your beloved.

Sound

The soft, sensual sounds of lips touching lips and tongues playing with each other can be exciting; sighs and moans of pleasure are very erotic. Your sounds let your lover know you are enjoying his or her kisses, but don't go overboard. Slurping and loud smacking sounds can be kiss "busters."

Touch

A kiss can be electrifying because the lips and tongue are dense with nerves and, therefore, very sensitive. When lips meet lips, they should be soft and kissably moist. Apply lip balm, petroleum jelly, or other lip moisturizer daily, especially during the summer months or if you tend to have dry, chapped lips. Don't get so wrapped up in the lip lock that you forget to use your hands to touch each other's body and face.

Kissing Techniques

To be truly sensational, kissing requires the active participation of both people, and it must be reciprocal, with each person fully participating and responding to the actions of the other. Most kisses are variations of two basic techniques: kissing with mouths closed and with mouths open.

Kisses should initially be soft and gentle. Begin with the mouth closed or only slightly parted. The muscles of your face and mouth must be relaxed. It might help to think of kissing as something you do with your mouth instead of primarily lips. Tightly pursed and puckered lips aren't kissable and make you seem like a novice. Relaxing your lips allows you to make contact with more of your partner's mouth.

Lightly brush your lips across your partner's lips, then plant soft, gentle kisses fully against his mouth. Add variety by gently kissing your partner's cheeks, nose, brow, eyelids, ears, and neck, observing which areas seem to be most pleasurable to him. If he enjoys something in particular, he'll likely reciprocate your kisses in a like fashion. Vary things a little more by pressing your mouth a little more firmly against his or for longer periods of time. Add a little nibbling action, gently tasting his lips.

For some couples, this will be the extent of their kisses. For many women "dry" kissing is much more romantic and loving than tongue kissing; for some, "tonguing" is distasteful. Others will venture further to the more erotic soul, tongue, or French-kissing techniques. If you are interested in further adventures, read on.

Return to his lips, this time with your mouth slightly parted. Now use the tip of your tongue to lightly lick his lips. He's not an ice-cream cone, so don't lap at him. Just allow your tongue to trace just inside his lips, starting from the corner of his lower lip, tasting your way across to the opposite side, and then across his upper lip. Go slowly, observing his response. If he's new at this game, urge him to relax and enjoy this kissing experiment.

Take his lower lip into your mouth, exploring the outer and inner surfaces of his lip with your tongue, and sucking very gently. He will most likely do the same to your upper lip. Then switch, taking his upper lip into your mouth, offering him your lower lip.

After you've enjoyed each other's lips for a while, venture a little deeper, allowing your tongue to enter his mouth. Your tongues should flirt, chase, and explore each other. Keep your mouth and tongue relaxed; don't tense the muscles up. This is a dance, not a wrestling match. Don't try to force your tongue deeply into his mouth or down his throat. Some men make that mistake, using their tongues the way they would use their penis, forcing their stiff tongues deeply into their partner's mouths. If he does this to you, pull away and start again. He'll soon get the hint. Also avoid sucking too vigorously on his tongue, or he may feel like he stuck his tongue into a vacuum cleaner. Likewise, a tongue that darts around rapidly with no direction doesn't have a chance to enjoy the sensual pleasures of the mouth. No one likes a dead tongue, either. If you just let it lie there like a piece of salami all the time, you won't be much fun to kiss.

Slowly explore his whole mouth: Brush your tongue along his teeth and gums—unless he suffers from tooth decay, in which case you probably don't want to kiss him anyway. You can even explore the roof of his mouth and the inside of his cheeks, allowing him to explore your mouth as well.

Get passionate, but don't get too carried away. Don't open your mouth too wide while you're kissing; you don't want his entire mouth between your lips. There are few things worse than pulling away from a kiss and finding that your face is wet from nose to chin. Also, please try not to drool or drip. Your kisses should be moist but not sloppy, so as you kiss, *swallow*. If you can't seem to swallow while you're kissing, pull away or move to another kissable area periodically to give yourself time to swallow.

As you get more intimate with each other and gain more confidence with your technique, you can change things up a little by altering the speed, pressure, depth, and intensity of your kisses as you nibble, suck, lick, press, and rub. You may even try lightly biting your lover's lips or tongue. Ask permission, or at least warn him or her before you do it the first time. It may be erotic for some people, but it may send chills of fear down the spine of others. As a medical student, I heard about a woman who lost her tongue when her partner had a seizure while they were French kissing. That was enough to keep my tongue in my mouth for a long time—but not forever!

The keys to being a great kisser are an obvious love of the art of kissing and creativity. You also need to communicate. When you try a new technique with your partner, let it be a pleasant surprise, but don't spring too much on him too soon. You don't have to explain in step-by-step detail what you're going to do; you'd risk taking the fun and spontaneity out of the experience. Just give him that special look and whisper in his ear: "Let's try something . . ." Then pay careful attention to his response to your kissing "experiments." Follow his cues and try to adjust your new moves to his rhythm and style.

Let your partner know that you are enjoying sharing the innocent but erotic pleasure of kissing with him—or that you want to. But what if you still hate the way your partner kisses? Don't discard him right away; he's likely to improve with more practice. Try this by way of instruction: Ask him to kiss you the way he likes to be kissed; then ask if you can kiss him the way that you like to be kissed. After this exercise, he should have a clear picture of what turns you on—as should you of him.

Keeping It Safe

Kissing can bring you great joy, but like all things pleasurable, there are risks. Don't lock lips if either of you has a cold sore near or on your lips— not even a quick peck. The herpes simplex virus can be transmitted during kissing of any kind. Likewise, the viruses that cause mononucleosis (kissing disease), hepatitis, the common cold and flu, and bacteria can be transmitted while tongue-kissing an infected partner.

Chapter 7
Delicacy #2: Touch

Think back to the last time you had sex. How much time did the two of you spend touching each other? Quite a bit you say? Okay, suppose I said that touching the breasts or genitals doesn't count. A different story? The truth is that most of us don't spend enough time appreciating the power and pleasure of touch. As with kissing, women often complain that the longer a relationship lasts, the less time is spent on the "little things" like touch. There's less hand-holding, fewer caresses, no spontaneous hugs. Touch becomes relegated to the category of "foreplay" or a preliminary step to "real sex"—intercourse. In fact, many couples never touch each other unless it's a prelude to or part of sex. Of those who do, some spend less than a minute touching each other before moving to the sex organs.

But touch isn't a "little thing." As infants, we crave touch; it's almost as necessary to human growth and development as food. The craving doesn't go away when we're adults. The gentle touch of another human being is comforting and healing: It has been suggested that being touched frequently may help you live a longer and happier life. It makes you feel better in the short term, too. Touch has been shown to decrease the stress level, blood pressure, and pulse rate of both the provider and the receiver, and it causes the brain to release "feel-good" chemicals called *endorphins*. It can be relaxing, affectionate, or sexually stimulating—or all three at the same time.

Touch Types

Touch can be as simple as putting your hand on another person. Even if you don't move another muscle, you're capable of sending tremendous energy and warmth through your hands to your partner's body. There are many ways to touch, and when you're sharing touch with your partner, it is important to try a variety of different types. Some of the touch techniques below can get you started. Remember, as you transition from one type of touch to another, to avoid sudden, jarring movements. Movements should be smooth and flowing, and your hands should stay relaxed.

Stroking

Your whole hand moves across his skin and body, as if you were bathing him or rubbing lotion into his skin. Strokes should always be gentle though you can vary the pressure you apply from a light stroke to a deep-tissue stroke. Strokes can be small or large. You can move in any number of directions or trace imaginary figures on the body of your partner. You can give a very pleasurable massage using stroking touch only.

Raking

Using the tips of your fingers and your nails, move your fingers across the body as if you were scratching him. The movements can be very light or you can apply heavier pressure. Always be aware of the body cues given by your partner as you rake his skin. If you have long nails, use extra caution to prevent injury.

Kneading

Handle the skin and tissue as you would if you were kneading dough: Pick up and squeeze the skin and underlying tissue between your thumbs and fingers. Kneading is wonderful in areas of the body with large muscles like the back, upper arms, thighs, and buttocks.

Percussion

Percussion is a light tapping movement. One method of percussion consists of lightly and rapidly tapping the skin with the side of your little fingers. Or you can cup your hands and gently use the entire cupped hand to rapidly tap the skin and underlying tissue. Be careful that you don't tap too hard or your partner might become tense rather than relaxed. Percussion is best used on areas with large muscles, so avoid the stomach and bony areas.

Vibrating

Your hands are placed on your partner's body and moved very rapidly up and down or side to side, creating a vibratory sensation.

Pinching

Yes, a pinch can be pleasurable if done carefully and lovingly. Gently pull the skin up between your thumb and first finger.

Getting Started

Without question, touch can intensify and electrify your lovemaking, but it doesn't have to be sexual to be pleasurable. Touch is a way to communicate. Consider the message you would receive if your lover gently stroked your face while gazing into your eyes. With a touch like that, who needs words? Try it. Take turns with your partner, touching each other all over and in all kinds of loving ways, but ignore each other's genitals and don't cap off the experience with intercourse. It's likely that you will find it a very satisfying experience even without sexual intercourse.

Some people shy away from touch because they associate it with elaborate massage and fear that they will not be "good" at it. But there really is no magic formula to touching. You don't need a diploma from the local massage school; all you need is your hands and the desire to please and be pleased through touch.

Bathing

For a nice, clean way to get more loving touch into your love life, try a sensual bath. Prepare a tub of warm water for your lover with bubbles, bath salts, flower petals, or essential oils. Using a soft cloth or sponge or your hands, simply wash his entire body. Be gentle, as if you were bathing a baby. Don't linger at his genitals or you may never make it to the remainder of the touching session. He'll surely enjoy the feeling of warm water running down his body and the silky feeling of soap on his skin, but you should pay attention to those senses and enjoy them as well. Have him step out before the water gets too cold, then wrap him in a warm towel, dry him slowly and carefully, and rub him down with body oil or lotion. If you don't have time for a full-fledged bath, hop into the shower with your lover and enjoy touching each other under the cascade of water.

Massage

A good way to really spend time touching is to offer your partner a massage. He'll surely appreciate the relaxing benefits, and you'll have an opportunity to get to know every inch of his body. If you're the masseuse, you direct the type of touch and the duration. You get to decide how far the touching goes.

Pick a warm, comfortable room where you won't be disturbed. You need to have enough space for your partner to stretch out completely and for you to move around him. Soft lighting helps set a relaxing mood, and soft music can help create a wonderful relaxing environment but is not necessary. If you are going to perform the massage on the bed, make sure you cover your sheets with a large soft towel or a fabric that you don't mind staining with oil.

A good massage oil is a necessity. You can purchase one with or without scent. Be aware that if you purchase massage oil with a fragrance, there is the possibility that your partner won't like the scent or that one of you may have an allergic reaction. Test it on a small area of skin prior to using it for massage. Almond oil is a traditional favorite, but any light cooking oil, such as sesame oil, can be used.

Warm the oil by placing the container in a bowl of warm water prior to beginning the massage, and keep it within easy reach throughout the massage. A plastic squeeze bottle provides easy, mess-free access to the oil. If working on a hard, flat surface, you can place the warm oil in a shallow bowl for easy access.

Massage is best done with your partner completely nude. This will allow you to reach every inch of his skin, and you won't have to work around clothing. For his privacy or warmth, you can drape a warm towel or light blanket over half of his body and adjust it as you proceed with the massage.

Touching

Once you have a comfortable space arranged you can prepare to touch your partner. Make sure your hands are clean and that you've filed or clipped sharp or ragged nails. Be aware of any rough calluses; they can give interesting sensations when massaging some areas of the body but can be uncomfortable when touching others. Use hand cream to smooth out those rough dry areas in advance. Warm your hands by soaking them in warm water or briskly rubbing them together.

The keys to the art of touch are gentleness, slow pace, and communication with your partner. Ask him to let you know through nonverbal cues what he finds pleasurable and what he doesn't, and remember to do the same when it is your turn to receive. You should not talk too much during a massage; focus on the feelings. Vary your strokes. Some are slow, some fast, some soft, and some firm and probing. Remember the "touch types" from the previous section. Try not to lose contact with your lover's skin once you begin touching: Keep one hand on his body even when applying more oil. A trick is to pour the oil into your upturned hand as it rests on your partner's body. If the oil is in a bowl, rest one hand on your partner's body while you dip the other into the oil.

Procedures

You can begin a massage with any part of the body. If your lover is feeling a lot of tension in his shoulders, you may want to start there. Or maybe his feet are tired and achy. Start wherever seems most appropriate and most appreciated. Just don't start with the genitals or the "massage" may turn quickly into sex. Remember that you're trying to focus on loving touch, not on getting to intercourse.

Back

We generally hold lots of tension in our backs, so massaging there can ease that tension and spread a sense of relaxation throughout the rest of the body. Don't be insulted if your partner falls asleep during this massage; it is a sign that you have given him the wonderful gift of total relaxation.

Your partner should lie on his stomach with his arms relaxed a few inches from his sides. He may want a soft, flattish pillow under his head for comfort. You can stand or kneel at his side or you may also choose to kneel, straddling his buttocks. Be sure not to sit or lean on his body during the massage. Begin by placing one warm hand on the center of his upper back between his shoulder blades and resting the other lightly in the center of his lower spine just above his buttocks. Remember, there is no pressure to "do it right." Any loving touch is likely to make your partner feel pampered and special. Focus on the pleasure that you wish to share and, as you breath out, send your feelings of love or admiration through your hands and into the body of your lover. As you breathe, your partner will feel warm energy radiating from your stationary hands.

Turn one of your hands over and pour the warm massage oil into your palm. Now spread the oil over half of his back by sliding the palm of your hand from one end of his back to the other. Repeat the oil application on the other half of his back with your other hand. Use plenty of oil, especially if his back is hairy, so that your hands glide effortlessly over his skin. Once his skin has been well oiled, you can begin to experiment with a variety of modalities of touch. Remember to add more oil as needed as you proceed with the massage.

Using your fingertips only, lightly stroke his back. Begin with one hand at the top of his back and slowly stroke down to the bottom. As one hand reaches the bottom of the back, begin at the top of his back with the other hand. Alternate your hands, creating a gently relaxing effect.

Now both hands should meet at the base of his spine. The hands are flat, palms down, and fingers together. With your hands on either side of his spine, slide them both up his back to his neck, using a moderate amount of pressure. At his neck, slide your hands out over his shoulders, and then down along his sides with your fingertips pointing toward the bed or table. Slide your fingers back up to the center of his lower spine and start over. Slowly repeat this stroke at least ten times with varying amounts of pressure.

When your hands meet at the base of his spine, slide only one hand up to his shoulder; as that hand starts to slide back down his back, begin to stroke up with the other hand. The hands move like a seesaw, alternating up and down both sides of his spine. Start slowly and speed up slightly before moving on to another type of touch.

The back is a great area to knead. Kneading the back muscles promotes relaxation and decreases muscle tension. Knead the large muscles of the upper and lower back, but not directly over the spine.

Follow kneading with additional gentle stroking. Make circles of varying sizes using the fingers and then the palms of your hands. Place your thumbs on either side of the spine. Make small circular movements with your thumbs as your hands move alongside the spine.

Rake or scratch his back using long strokes along the full length of his back.

Place one hand on top of the other and use your body weight to slide the hands up the middle of the back from his buttocks to his neck and back again.

Standing or kneeling at his side, place the ball of your hands at his spine with your fingertips facing the bed or table. Slide one hand down his side, toward the bed, and then back up again. As that hand is sliding back up his side, move the other hand down his side toward the bed. Alternate the hands up and down as they move along the spine.

Still by his side, slide your hands together from the base of one side of his back to the base of the other side of his back. Your strokes should be long, smooth, and continuous across the full expanse of his back.

You can help relax tense muscles by using percussion on the upper and lower back with the side of your little fingers or your cupped hands. Keep it gentle and do not percuss directly over the spine.

Vibratory touch feels great on the upper back and shoulders. Complete your massage of his back by gently stroking the entire back with the lightest touch of your fingers.

Back of Arms

Remembering not to take your hands off your partner, add more oil and proceed to his arms. You should move your hands smoothly, in long, gentle strokes from his back to his shoulders and down his arms to his hands. The shoulders often hold lots of tension, so they should be stroked and kneaded individually for a while. Percussion also works well here. Place one hand on either side of his arm, encircling it as much as possible, and slide your hands up and down the entire arm. Gentle kneading with the thumb and two fingers feels great as you move up and down the back of the arms. When ready to move on, slide your hands up the arms, across the shoulders, and down the back to the buttocks.

Buttocks

The buttock muscles are often neglected, but they can be quite tense and in dire need of attention and relaxation. Because they are large muscles, any modality of touch works well. Begin with long, firm strokes down the middle of his buttocks and up the sides. Change the direction of the strokes as well as the speed and pressure. Kneading and percussion should be mixed with a variety of different stroking movements and be followed by light circular stroking. Vibration creates a very erotic sensation when applied to the buttocks.

Be aware that some people find buttock massage to be uncomfortable. Look for cues from your partner. If he stiffens up, it may be a sign to move on to the next area.

Back of Legs

As you complete your buttock massage, slide one hand down each leg to the feet and back up again, then down the inner thighs and legs to his ankles and up the outer legs, thighs, and buttocks. Reverse direction by sliding down the outer leg and up the inner leg. Your upward movements should be firm; downward strokes light. Complete the circuit several times before concentrating on one leg at a time.

Starting with one leg, place both hands on either side of it and stroke the length of his leg, starting at the ankle and sliding up to the buttocks and back down again. Repeat this stroke several times. From the side and starting at the ankle, knead the entire leg. Do the other leg.

NOTE: Do not massage your partner's legs if he has *phlebitis* (inflammation of his veins), swelling, skin irritation, or clots in his blood vessels.

When you finish the leg massage, slide your hands up from the ankles, up the legs, over the buttocks, up the back, across the shoulders, and down the arms to the hands. Now have your partner turn over to his back while you shift your body so that you are positioned at his head and facing him. Should your partner have an erection at this point, ignore it. There are other body parts screaming for attention.

Head and Scalp

Place your hands on either side of your lover's face. (Don't use oil for this part.) Continue to breathe slowly and deeply. Begin to massage his scalp by making circular motions covering the sides, back, and top of his head. Keeping your movements slow, soothing, and gentle, bring your hands back to the sides of his head and lightly massage his temples using the same small circular motions. Now slide your hands down the sides of his face and behind his neck. The neck is often a site of significant muscle tension, so spend as much time as needed stroking the back of his neck from his shoulders to the base of his skull. Make long, gentle strokes, alternating your hands up and down. Slide your hands down his neck and onto his chest.

Chest and Abdomen

Apply oil to your upturned hand. Slide your hands gently along his chest from his neck to just above his pubic area, spreading the oil. Using only your fingers at first, gently stroke the entire expanse of the chest and abdomen. Then, using your entire hands, slide your hands down the chest and over the abdomen. When you reach the pubic area, slide your hands out to the side and slide up the sides of the abdomen and chest. Repeat several times.

Use the entire hands with fingers together to make circular strokes of

A Little-Known Fact:
Male Breast Cancer

One percent of all breast cancer occurs in men. The incidence increases as men age. Here is how to check for breast cancer in a man. As you slide your hands across his chest and tweak his nipples, be aware of any lumps or thickening of the breast tissue as well as any discharge from his nipples. Bring any unusual findings to his attention and encourage him to see a physician.

moderate pressure over the chest and lighter pressure over the abdomen. Knead the muscles of the upper chest and shoulders, then move outward, stroking the arms and hands again.

Front of Arms and Hands

Massage the arms, one at a time, beginning with long flowing strokes from the shoulder all the way to his hands. Alternate your strokes, using one hand to stroke up as the other strokes down on either side of the arm. Place one hand on either side of the arm and make long, firm strokes from the wrist to the shoulders and back down. Imagine you are pulling the tension out of his arms.

Knead the arm muscles as you move from the shoulder to the hands by placing both hands around the arm and making circular movements with your thumbs. When you reach the hand, use your thumbs to massage his palm and the back of his hand. Hold his hands and stroke them from the wrist to the fingers, then stroke the sides of each finger separately, pulling gently as you go.

Slide your hands up the arms, across his shoulders, and continue along his chest and stomach.

Front of Legs

The legs have large muscles that are used constantly and need some TLC. Pour oil into your upturned hand and, using the palm of your hand, spread it along the front of one leg then the other, stroking him from his feet up to his groin. Use long strokes, then short strokes, and vary the pressure. Stroke the outside of the legs as you slide up and the inside of the legs on the way down. Knead the muscles of the entire upper legs. Percussion movement can also be used on the upper thighs, but avoid percussion over the bony area of the shins. Make light feathery strokes down the legs to the feet.

Feet

The feet are the most overlooked part of the body, but they take a beating and can always use some extra care. Using lots of oil, take one foot in both hands and gently stroke it from the ankle over the top and sides of the foot. Cup the heel of the left foot in your left hand. Make circular movements using your thumb to massage just below the inside ankle and your fingers to massage below the outside ankle. Then use the thumb of your right hand to knead the heel of the foot. Massage each toe individually between your thumb and two fingers, pulling gently as you reach the tip of each toe. Now switch to the right foot, using the right hand, and do the same.

You can end the massage by making long feathery finger strokes from his feet up to his neck and back several times. If you so desire, you can continue to his genitals for erotic massage play.

Total Body-to-Body Massage

Another way to end a massage session is with full-body massage. This can be a lot of fun even if a little messy. Spread lots of oil over your chest, abdomen, and the front of your legs and arms. Do the same for your partner. Now slide your body over the front of your partner's body. Slide up and down and side to side. Make large circles with your body. Turn him over and slide over the full expanse of his back, buttocks, and legs.

Genital Massage

It's pretty easy to learn to give a good "hand job." Once you learn the basic techniques, you can develop your own signature style, practicing what is most erotic and exciting for your partner.

The very best way to learn what your partner loves is to watch him masturbate. You can make mental notes of where he places his hand, his strokes, speed, rhythm, and even the amount of pressure that he likes. If he's not into show-and-tell, you'll have to experiment with him. Vary your technique and note what seems to give him the most pleasure.

The most comfortable position for you to be in while giving a hand job is kneeling between his legs while he lies on his back. If you want to be massaged at the same time, a side-to-side position is best, but for now you want to put all your attention on pleasuring him. Choose a water-based lubricant and warm it by rubbing it between your hands before you touch his genitals. If you won't be using a condom or having vaginal intercourse later, you can use a longer-lasting oil-based lubricant.

Begin by gently placing your hand, palm down, on his penis. Just let it rest there for a while and don't move. Trust me: He'll notice the natural heat and energy from your hand and will twitch with anticipation of what is to come. If he likes to have his scrotum touched, slide your other hand down to his scrotum and gently cover his scrotum with your hand. As he warms up, start to lightly glide your hand along the length of the underside of his penis.

Using your dominant hand, grasp the shaft of the penis in your hand. Stroke only the shaft of the penis up and down. After a while lengthen your stroke, starting at the base of the penis and continuing up and past the head and back down again. Change the pressure and speed of your strokes. To make this stroke even better, gently twist your hand in one direction on the way up and over the head and in the other direction on the way down.

Resume the up-and-down strokes, but this time as you reach the head on the upstroke, twist the palm of your hand completely over the head of his penis and then continue with the downstroke. Repeat this stroke for a while before moving on. Watch his expressions—and the reaction of his penis—to see what he likes.

Cup the head of the penis in the palm of your hand and, with your fingers pointing down, grip the sides of the shaft and rotate your palm in one direction and then the other. Make sure the palm of your hand is well lubricated. While stroking his penis with one hand, you can use your other hand to massage his scrotum, perineum, inner thigh, or anus. You can also alternate stroking his penis with oral pleasuring.

Take it slowly and observe what seems to be getting the biggest rise out of your partner. Experiment and vary your movement. Remember that stimulating the same area in the exact same way for prolonged periods of time may lead to a numb feeling and a very limp penis.

It Takes Two

There are many genital massage techniques using two hands. Start by grasping the penis with both lubricated hands, one on top of the other, then moving both hands up the shaft and head of the penis and back down again. Your partner will have the sensation of thrusting deeply into a long, tight vagina. Vary this stroke by twisting one hand in one direction and the other in the opposite direction as you move up and down.

Grasp the head of the penis with both hands. Place one thumb on each side of the frenulum. Now move your thumbs up and down in opposite directions along the frenulum, varying the speed as you notice what seems to be giving him the most pleasure.

Place your palms on both sides of the penis. Now alternate rubbing your hands up and down or back and forth along the length and head of the penis.

Grasp the head of the penis with your right hand and slide down the shaft. As you reach the base of the penis, grasp the head with your left hand and slide down the shaft as your right hand releases and goes back up to the head. Repeat this "milking" motion, alternating your hands. Reverse, grasping the penis at the base with your right hand and slide your hand up the shaft and head. As you reach the head, grasp the penis at the base with your left hand and slide up the shaft.

Receiving Sensual Massage

Once you've practiced giving your partner a massage, you've not only touched him in a loving, relaxing, and sensuous way, you've also shown him what to do when it's your turn. No matter how proficient he is, the massage won't be a great one unless you're receptive. Keep these things in mind:

- Relax and give his hands your full attention.

- Let him know what feels good and what is missing the mark.

- Make sure you have plenty of water-based lubricant for genital massage.

- Allow him to watch you masturbate to get the best view of what turns you on.

- Don't be shy. Use your hands to guide his hands to the right spot, the right stroke, and the right pressure. Remember, you deserve to be pleasured!

- Don't just lie there. Move your hips to assure that your most sensitive areas are stroked.

The biggest mistake that men make is to rub too hard and too fast. Again, communication is key. If it doesn't feel good, let him know either verbally or nonverbally by pulling away and directing his hand. If his goal is to please you, he will welcome your input.

If his fingernails are causing a burning sensation in your delicate tissues, stop. It is better to stop now and bring out the clippers than to suffer with a sore, injured vulva and vagina for the next few days.

Loving Women

Manual Sex Play: Using Your Hands

If you've spent some time masturbating, learning to lead your partner into a state of ecstasy should be easy. But I'll be the first to tell you that every woman is different, and it is best to find out what type of manual stimulation she likes before making love.

The best way to learn her preferences is to ask her, or ask her to masturbate in front of you. Watch carefully to see where she puts her fingers, how many fingers she uses, how she moves her fingers, and the speed of her movements. Place your hand on top of hers to get a feel for the pressure that she uses when she self-loves. Or you can ask her to place your hand where she likes to be stimulated and move your hand in the way that gives her pleasure. And since you may want her to reciprocate, show her how you self-stimulate.

Before you even think about touching a woman's delicate tissues, you need to get prepared. First, you must make sure that your hands and nails are clean to prevent vaginal infections. Cut and trim your nails. If you have just spent a fortune on 3-inch tips, you might consider a different method of giving her pleasure. I have treated many women with tears, cuts, and scrapes from lovely acrylic nail tips. If you can't get rid of the tips, then cover your nails with cotton balls and put on latex gloves.

Lubrication is a must during manual sex play. Rubbing a dry clitoris with a dry finger will cause burning, swelling, and discomfort that can last for hours or days. Even if she feels wet, water-based lubricants give a sensuous feel and help to protect the skin of her labia and clitoris. Choose a lubricant that does not have an unpleasant taste in case you want to combine manual and oral sex play.

There are many positions for manual sex play. Try asking your partner to lie on her back while you kneel or lie beside her, or you can kneel between her legs facing her.

Don't go right for her clitoris during manual sex play; work up to it. You've got time, so start by touching, stroking, and massaging her entire body. Feel the texture and warmth of her skin and let her know how good she feels.

Spend some time massaging and stroking her lower abdomen, inner thighs, and buttocks. Slowly start to move your hands in toward her mons and labia. Begin with a very light touch that just barely brushes her skin. Now take your whole hand and cover her vulva, allowing the warmth and energy from your hand to move through her genitals. Now move your hand slowly up and down, then in circles. Keep the pressure light unless she asks for more.

Use two or three fingers to trace her labia majora from top to bottom. Using the same motion, trace her labia minora from the bottom of one, over the hood of her clitoris, and down the other. Circle the entrance to her vagina, but don't enter yet. Slide your finger along the space between her labia majora and labia minora and along the sides of her clitoris.

Some women like direct stimulation of the clitoris and some don't. Ask her. If she does want to have her clitoris stroked, use one or two fingers and starting at the top of the shaft of the clitoris (at the mons) slide your finger down over the shaft and to the vagina. Now slide your fingers back up again. When you slide up, do not curl your fingers in or you might injure the clitoris with your nails. Spend some time with the up-and-down movement, then vary the direction from side to side to circular (large circles and small circles). Vary the speed but keep the pressure light until she asks for more. If your partner likes to have her vagina stroked as well, you can slide your fingers from her mons, over her clitoris, and into her vagina. The key to good manual stimulation is variety. If you use one stroke in the same spot for too long, the clitoris (or labia) may become numb.

G-Spot Massage

The G-spot is an exciting area of exploration. Many women get a great deal of pleasure from the stimulation of this sensitive area on the front wall of their vaginas. Others don't find it exciting at all. Still others don't even know they have it. Talk to your partner to find out what she knows about this potentially sensitive part of her body. If she's willing, the two of you can go on a journey to find it.

Again, make sure your nails are well trimmed and that you have lots of lubricant on hand. Stimulate her labia and clitoris before beginning the G-spot massage so that she is fully aroused. Slowly insert one or two fingers into her vagina with your palm facing up and press them against the front wall of her vagina as you move them in and out. Each time you pull your fingers back, curl them as if beckoning someone to "come here." As you stroke her, you may notice a small area midway between her cervix and pubic bone that feels like a small lump. This is her G-spot, and it will increase in size as you stimulate it. You can vary the movement of your fingers on her G-spot: Try in-and-out, zigzag, side-to-side, or circular motions. Add to her pleasure by placing your thumb on her clitoris and massaging it at the same time you massage her G-spot.

Keeping It Safe

Though the chances of getting a sexually transmitted disease through manual stimulation are low, it is possible. Bacteria and viruses in her vaginal secretions can be transmitted through small cracks in your skin. So if you are not sure about the health status of your partner, use latex gloves or a finger cot (a latex sleeve that covers one finger) to protect your hand or fingers from her vaginal secretions. Be sure to change the gloves before touching your own genitals.

Chapter 8

Delicacy #3: Outercourse

When you have outercourse with your partner, you're stimulating each other's genitals without actual penetration into the vagina. If you've never tried it as a variation on your sexual activities, you've missed a real treat. Many women have found that they achieve orgasm more often with outercourse than intercourse. And with the right moves, your partner will find it irresistible.

Getting Started

Begin by lying on your back and apply a water-based lubricant to your labia, clitoris, and inner thighs. Better yet, have your partner do it. Lubricate the head and shaft of his penis. If you have thick or coarse pubic hair, make sure you lubricate well.

Your partner lowers himself on top of you. Separate your legs just enough to allow his penis to slide between your thighs and up against your vulva and clitoris. You can spread the labia to gain better access to your clitoris if you like. Now close your legs, trapping the penis between your thighs and vulva. As he thrusts, elevate your hips, contract your pelvic floor muscles, and press your clitoris against his penis. As he withdraws, slide your clitoris down against his penis. Try circular motions to get a good clitoral massage. Use your strong inner thigh muscles to massage the penis and to help pull it firmly against your most sensitive spots. At no time does the penis enter your vagina, however.

Variations

Outercourse can also be performed while standing with your back against a wall. If he's much taller than you are, he'll need to stoop or you'll have to tiptoe or both. That may not be as comfortable for either of you as lying down, but it's worth a try.

For a different experience, try outercourse from the rear. Lie on your stomach after applying lubricant between your thighs and buttocks and on your vulva. He lies on top and slides his penis between your buttocks, being careful not to enter your anus or vagina. As he strokes forward, you arch your back and swing your buttocks up and back toward his penis. His penis will slide down the space between your buttocks and over the opening of your vagina. If he is longer than average, he may even massage the head of your clitoris with the head of his penis. Use your well-developed gluteal (buttock) muscles to squeeze and massage the length of his penis as he withdraws and your pelvis rocks forward.

Keeping It Safe

During outercourse, the penis never enters the vagina, but that doesn't mean that you don't need contraception. If he ejaculates anywhere near the vagina it is possible for the sperm to swim up and conception to occur. Likewise, it is possible to get a sexually transmitted disease without entering your vagina. I've seen many "virgins" who had herpes, warts, or other sexually transmitted infections after outercourse. As with any other sex act, use the proper protection if you're not sure of your partner's health status.

When you're performing outercourse from the back, the penis does slide along the outside of the anus, so it is important to wash the area before you begin and to wash the vaginal opening thoroughly after this experience to decrease your risks of a vaginal infection. Follow the usual safe-sex practices to avoid pregnancy and sexually transmitted infections (STIs).

Chapter 9

Delicacy #4: Oral Sex

The first time someone gently guided my head down to his penis I wasn't sure what I was supposed to do with it. Should I sniff it, lick it, suck it, chew it, or bite it? I didn't even feel comfortable looking at it, much less putting it in my mouth. But there I was, up close and personal. I decided to give it a few quick licks and was surprised and hurt by his shrieks of laughter.

—Anonymous

Fellatio, also known as "giving head," giving a "blow job" (though it is unusual for anyone to actually blow on the penis), and "going down" on the penis, is one of the most misunderstood sexual acts. Because you stimulate a man's penis with your mouth rather than your vagina, some people don't view fellatio as "real" sex. In fact some young couples have turned to fellatio as a substitute for intercourse; they feel that it allows them to explore their sexuality without actually "doing it." The fear of pregnancy and sexually transmitted diseases has also helped increase the popularity of fellatio. You can't get pregnant from giving a blow job, but it's important to remember that sexually transmitted diseases, including HIV infections, can be transmitted through oral sex. So even oral sex must be practiced safely.

If you are a woman who already loves giving head, reading this section may help you learn new techniques. If your man likes oral stimulation, you can give him the ultimate pleasure by learning how to perform masterful fellatio.

Conversely, if the thought of a blow job makes you gag, you shouldn't feel obligated. Remember, you are in charge of what you do sexually. Fellatio is definitely not for everyone, and if you're uncomfortable doing it, you're not likely to give yourself or your partner much pleasure. Likewise, if you are doing it only because you feel an obligation to do it, or if you feel that he is forcing or coercing you to do it, you are more likely to feel resentment than pleasure, and that will only increase your distaste for the practice.

By the same token, if you're just unsure about it, give it a shot before you make a final judgment. If you learn good technique and have a sensitive, gentle partner to practice on, you may find that you enjoy it more than you imagined. With a little practice, you may find that it is a very erotic, intimate, and intensely personal experience.

Men love receiving oral sex because they are able to just lie back and enjoy without any performance anxiety. They can watch, too, and since they are the stars of the show, it's a better turn-on than any porno flick. Women get their own sense of pleasure from fellatio. "I feel powerful when I give a blow job," one of my colleagues told me. "At no other time do I feel such complete control of my partner's pleasure." She shares the sentiments of many other women who like the feeling of power they get from having his most prized possession between their lips. Some women find it very arousing to watch their partners enjoy their oral mastery.

Learning Oral Technique

If you've never performed fellatio before, you might want to practice all of the moves and techniques described on an inanimate object before introducing them to your lover. My suggestion is to use a dildo. If you don't have one, you can purchase an inexpensive one in a sex shop or discreetly on the Internet. If you don't feel comfortable buying a dildo, substitute a clean peeled cucumber or a plus-sized carrot. Of course, if your lover is patient and is game to be a guinea pig, you can certainly practice on him.

Whatever or whomever you practice on, remember that every man is different and likes different things. The best way to find out what your partner likes is to ask him, but don't be surprised if he finds it difficult to describe in words what turns him on about oral sex. He might be better able to tell you what he particularly likes or dislikes while you are giving him oral stimulation. Try different things and watch his verbal and non-verbal cues. Often it will become obvious what he really enjoys.

Get into Position

Before beginning to pleasure the penis, it's important to find a position that is comfortable for you and your partner. Perhaps the best position for oral sex is with him lying on his back and you kneeling between his legs facing him. If his penis angles tightly against his abdominal wall when it's erect, you may need to lean forward over his body to get the right angle; pulling the erect penis down toward you can be uncomfortable for him.

For variety, you can also try the following:

- He can lie on his back while you kneel at his side and bend over his genitals at an angle. You can place pillows under his buttocks to make it easier on your neck.

- Using pillows to support your neck, lie beside him with your head at the level of his penis.

- Lie on your back and let him straddle your chest on his knees, dangling his genitals from above. Women generally have less control in this position and find it to be the least pleasant.

- He can stand, sit in a chair, or sit on the edge of the bed while you kneel between his legs. Many women don't like this position, either, because it is the one most commonly assumed in porno movies. Some men love it for the same reason.

Getting to the Bottom of Oral Sex Myths

There are numerous myths and misconceptions about oral sex, many of which can interfere with your ability to enjoy the experience. Over the years I have heard a number of misconceptions about oral sex from my patients.

The penis is dirty.

The penis is covered with skin just like the rest of his body. As long as a man cleans himself daily, including under his foreskin if he is uncircumcised, his penis should be as clean as, say, his hands—or cleaner. It's certainly cleaner than his mouth, and there should be no offensive odor.

If you are concerned, share a bath or shower prior to oral sex. Soap him up, touch him all over, and rinse him off in a stream of warm water. You might even try giving a blow job while in the shower.

He might urinate in my mouth.

It is very difficult for a man with an erection to urinate, and he can't ejaculate and urinate at the same time.

I'll gag.

You can trigger a natural gag reflex when anything touches the back of your throat, but you can give a great blow job without the penis playing tag with your tonsils. If you keep it in the front of your mouth, relax, and breathe, you probably won't gag.

continued

He'll expect me to swallow.

Many women are concerned about the taste of semen and fear that it will be harmful if swallowed. First, you don't have to swallow. You can discreetly let his semen run out of your mouth and back down the shaft of his penis, or spit it out on the sheets. If you do choose to swallow, know that it is not harmful.

Only "bad girls" do it.

Get over it! There is no right or wrong way to express yourself sexually. More women are giving head than you think (as many as 75 percent according to *The Social Organization of Sexuality: Sexual Practices in the United States*). Increasing his pleasure will give you pleasure, and if you want him to perform *cunnilingus* (oral sex for women), it will encourage him to reciprocate.

I don't know how. I feel awkward.

You can do it! It just takes a little know-how—which you're getting plenty of just by reading this book.

It's not natural.

Who decides what's natural? Frankly anything that two adult people engage in and find mutually pleasurable is natural.

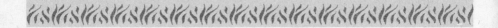

Give Him Some Lip

Fellatio involves the use of your lips, tongue, cheeks, and upper palate. The most important tool for giving head is your tongue, but the lips are very important, too. They spend most of their time covering your teeth to protect his penis. However, as you become more comfortable with fellatio, the lips can be used in more exciting ways.

You probably wouldn't like to have a lover immediately attack your clitoris when engaging in sex; likewise, you don't want to rush to the penis right away. To make things interesting and to keep him guessing about your plans, start with him lying on his stomach. With your hands, massage his buttocks, back, and neck, planting kisses along the way. Trace his spine with your tongue. To add spice, you might slip one hand between his legs and gently stroke his scrotum.

Now have him lie on his back, so you have access to his front. Start kissing his face, lips, neck, chest, and nipples. Suck gently on the nipples, using your tongue to increase stimulation. (Some men hate to have their nipples touched. If you haven't asked him, look for cues to determine whether he enjoys nipple play.) Alternate kissing and licking down the abdomen, including the navel. Spend a little time at the lower abdomen, between the navel and the pubic bone, an area that some men find super sensitive. As you near the genitals, brush your lips across the penis and scrotum ever so lightly.

Start again at the bottom, planting kisses from his toes to the inner thighs, licking and nibbling as you go along. The inner thighs tend to be sensitive in most, but not all, men; some men find the area ticklish. Underneath his scrotum and before you get to the anus, like you, he has a perineum, which is also sensitive so touch or lick in that area. As you move up to the penis, kiss and lick the entire surface of the scrotum. Some men love it when you gently take one testicle into your mouth. If he does, slide your tongue under his scrotum and lift it with your tongue. Some men hate to have their scrotum touched. Ask him what he likes.

The Main Event

You are now ready to give some attention to his penis. Begin with kissing and licking his entire penis. Make your tongue flat and lick the penis like an ice cream cone, starting at the base and working your way up to the head. Spend some time at the corona and the very sensitive frenulum, and lick back down again. The saliva you generate is a great lubricant and will make the rest of the blow job easier and more pleasurable. Be sure to lick him well to cover the entire shaft.

Hold the base of the penis with your hand and take the head of the penis into your mouth, leaving your lips slightly parted. Move your tongue in a circle around the head of the penis and let the front of your tongue stroke the underside of the penis and the soft underside of your tongue stroke the front of the penis. Breath through your mouth to enhance sensations. Now flick your tongue rapidly all over the surface of the glans and around the entire corona, lingering briefly at the frenulum. You should be able to tell by his reaction if this is what he likes. Don't be afraid to move your tongue in a different way that may be more comfortable for you or to try a technique he might suggest.

Take the head of the penis into your mouth and slide your mouth down the penis as far as you feel comfortable. (Watch your teeth. Most men hate the feel of teeth against their penis.) You should have practiced this with the dildo or cucumber beforehand so you know how far you can go before you start to gag. Slide his penis in and out of your mouth by moving your head up and down on it. Your lips should press lightly around the penis as you move; you can increase the pressure as he becomes more excited.

Giving Him More

Some men will be perfectly happy with this simple in-and-out movement of your mouth on the penis. But if you want him to be ecstatic, you need to learn more advanced moves and variations. It's important to vary your speed, lip pressure, amount of suction, and tongue moves while giving head. Be creative, experiment, and establish your own signature style. Here are some things to try. You can do them all in one session or spring them on him one at a time:

> Open your mouth wide and slide your tongue under his penis and push it up and down with your tongue—but watch your upper teeth if you have a very strong tongue. Breathe warm air through your mouth as you lift. He will be amazed at your strength.

- Place his penis in your mouth. Apply light pressure with your lips (while covering your teeth), and move your head from side to side, allowing the penis to move from one cheek to the other. Change the speed to add an interesting effect.

- Slide the penis into your mouth as far as you feel comfortable, stroking and massaging it with your tongue as you move your mouth up the shaft of the penis. Use slow movements with your flat tongue, then faster movements with your pointed tongue. When you reach the corona and frenulum, apply a little more pressure with your lips and let your tongue get a workout. Switch to massaging with your tongue on the downstroke or while moving up and down the shaft.

- Add interest by creating suction while moving your mouth up the shaft of the penis. Some men will like only the slightest hint of suction whereas others will crave a lot.

- Encircle the base of the penis with your thumb and as many fingers as you need, then as you move your mouth up and down the penis, let your fingers follow. (You will need lubrication, so apply saliva or a lubricant—try one that does not have a horrible taste.) He will have the sensation that he is deeper in your mouth as more of his penis is being stimulated.

- Lay his penis against his pubic bone or abdominal wall so that you're looking at the underside of the penis. Locate the corpus spongiosum and put your lips at the base of the penis with one of your lips on either side of it. Slide your lips up the shaft of the penis, keeping the spongiosum between your lips. As you slowly move up, suck and move your tongue along this sensitive area. Continue to the frenulum and tip of the penis, then go back down again.

- As you slide your mouth up the penis, move your head to the left side and then to the right side. You can vary this by twisting your head on the way down the shaft or in both directions.

⚲ "Snap" his head: After sliding your mouth up the shaft of the penis to the point just below the corona, apply more pressure with your lips and, with a light suction, pull your lips over the corona and head, creating a "snapping" sound.

⚲ Deep-throating requires taking the whole penis into your mouth and down your throat. This technique was made famous by the porno industry, but most women can't do it. You can give tremendous pleasure to your partner without stressing the back of your throat. If you want to try it, experiment with a dildo first to learn how to turn off your gag reflex. Because the tissues in the back of the throat are delicate and easily injured, you may find that you have a sore throat the day following deep-throating. Try gargling with warm salty water and suck on soothing throat lozenges for relief.

⚲ Assume the "sixty-nine" position, lying side by side or one on top of the other with your heads at each other's genitals. This position allows each of you to pleasure the other orally. It sounds great, but it is very hard to concentrate on pleasuring someone else when you are being pleasured. This is definitely a move for the experienced oral pleasurer.

⚲ For variety, place a small frozen melon ball in your mouth or drink something hot before placing the penis in your mouth. Sucking strong mints or mentholated cough drops before fellatio will also give him incredible sensations.

As you try any of these techniques, continue to pay attention to other parts of his body. Use your hands to stroke or gently cup his scrotum if that's what he likes. Massage the perineum between his scrotum and anus. Stroke his chest, nipples, thighs, or any other body part that he finds pleasurable. Let him know you are enjoying giving him pleasure.

And stay tuned to your partner. Look him in the eyes if you can. Read his body language, taking cues from his responses to tell you what seems to feel best and what doesn't work. Don't stop every minute and ask if you are doing a good job; if he seems to be enjoying what you are doing, keep going.

Other Considerations

The decision to swallow semen or not is all yours. If you don't want to, tell your partner so, and ask him to let you know when he is about to come so that you can finish him off with your hands. Using a flavored condom is another option.

Don't be surprised if you have very sore lips the day after performing fellatio the first few times. It takes practice to figure out just how to cover your teeth and just how much pressure to put on your lips.

Some men will start to thrust the penis deeply into your mouth as they become more excited. Some will even place their hands on your head and hold it down to try to get deeper into your mouth. If this makes you uncomfortable, let him know. You can also place your hand at the base of the penis to control how deeply the penis can enter your mouth.

Don't be surprised if your partner becomes "soft" while you're per-

Keeping It Safe

The risks of getting HIV during fellatio are less than during intercourse, but it pays to be safe. If you are not sure of his sexual health status, use a latex or polyurethane condom to decrease your risks of contracting not only HIV but also other sexually transmitted infections. Nonoxynol-9 tastes horrible, so you may prefer to use a condom without spermicide. Buy flavored latex condoms or add fat-free food products—jelly, syrup, honey—to the surface of an unflavored one. Whipped cream, which contains fat, may damage a latex condom, and edible condoms do not protect you at all from infections.

forming oral sex. It happens. If he seems to be enjoying what you're doing, keep at it. It won't be long before his erection returns.

At the time of this writing, oral sex and anal sex remain illegal in twelve states. In one state, sodomy between homosexual or heterosexual adults is punishable by as much as five years in jail. As long as you don't perform these or other sex acts in public, it is unlikely that these ancient laws will be enforced.

Loving Women: Cunnilingus

Perhaps the most intimate of sexual delicacies shared between women, oral sex can be intensely pleasurable for both the giver and the receiver. When you're giving oral sex, you are up close and personal with the most intimate part of your lover's body, and all your senses—sight, hearing, smell, taste, and touch—are stimulated.

It may be especially comforting to come face-to-face with your partner's genitals because everything is familiar. Just because she has the same anatomy, that doesn't mean that she likes the same things in the same way that you do. Every woman is different, and what turns you on may not do anything for her. It is always best to ask a new partner what she likes before making love or to move slowly at first and ask as you go along. One way to learn how to give her pleasure is to ask her to perform oral sex on you exactly the way that she likes to receive oral sex, and you can do the same.

The techniques of oral sex include kissing, licking, sucking, and careful, gentle nibbling. Study the kissing delicacy again; many of the techniques for kissing her mouth will also be effective when you are kissing her vulva. Don't expect to be perfect right away. It takes time to learn the preferences of your partner and all of her trigger points.

The Art of Cunnilingus

There are many positions for oral sex. Your partner can lie on her back while you lie on your stomach between her legs, or she can sit on the edge of a chair or bed while you kneel in front of her. You can lie on your back and your partner can straddle you, holding herself over your face. Or you

both can lie on your sides in the 69 position and give each other oral pleasure at the same time. Experiment and find the one that feels best for you
and your partner.

Good oral sex begins slowly and should not be rushed. Don't immediately rush to attack her clitoris. Begin by kissing, nibbling, and licking the
areas surrounding her genitals, her inner thighs, lower abdomen, and perineum. Come closer and plant kisses on her labia majora and mons.
Spread her labia and run your tongue in the grooves between her labia majora and labia minora, lick each lip, and gently suck them one at a time.
When you think she may be ready now for a little attention to her clitoris,
approach it slowly, flattening your tongue to lick her slowly from her
vagina up to and over the top of her clitoris and back down again. Spend
some time with this stroke, varying the speed and movement of your
tongue to keep it interesting.

When you are ready to focus on her clitoris, you might move your
tongue from side to side, up and down, or in circles around it. Vary the direction, speed, and pressure of your tongue and keep it moist; a dry tongue
can be abrasive. Don't jump from one thing to another too quickly. Try
one thing for a while to see how she responds to it before you go on to the
next technique.

Some women like direct stimulation of the clitoris and even enjoy having the hood pulled back to completely expose the glans during oral sex.
Sucking the clitoris can be exciting for some women. Try placing your lips
completely around her clitoris and sucking gently. While maintaining the
light suction, move your tongue slowly around her clitoris. For others, direct clitoral stimulation may be too much. They might get the most pleasure if you lick along the shaft and hood of the clitoris only. Whatever you
do, keep it light and gentle unless your partner requests stronger sucking
action.

The entrance to the vagina may be quite sensitive; inserting your tongue
as far as you can into her vagina can be a real turn-on. You can also give
her vagina some attention by inserting a finger or two into her vagina and
massaging her G-spot while your mouth is on her clitoris. Many women
like to have their breasts fondled while receiving oral sex, so try putting
your free hand to good use.

Cunnilingus: Getting as Good as You Give

If you enjoy performing oral sex on your man—and even if you don't—you'll probably love being licked by him. This practice is called *cunnilingus,* and many women find it not only pleasurable, but often the easiest route to orgasm as well. To get the most of this experience, try the following tips:

〰 If you take a bath or shower before cunnilingus, avoid using harsh deodorant soaps; the residue from them tastes terrible. Instead use a mild, unscented cleansing bar or cream and rinse thoroughly.

〰 Assist him by using your fingers to spread and hold your labia back to better expose your clitoris and vaginal opening. Likewise, if you desire a G-spot massage during oral pleasuring, guide one or two of his fingers to the spot.

〰 Choose a position that gives you the best range of motion, then move your hips to guide his tongue and lips to your most sensitive spots.

〰 If you're not the verbal type, then move those hips, moan, groan, sigh, or call out his name. If he is okay with it, you might even gently put your hands on the back of his head and direct him. But remember to let him breathe!

Communication with your partner is key. If you know what works for you, don't hesitate to tell him; if you're new to the game, then you'll have to give him clues as you go along. As in any sexual activity, if anything he does is painful, let him know. If he has a sore on or near his lips, avoid oral sex. The herpes virus that causes cold sores can be transmitted to your genitals.

Keeping It Safe

It's a myth that sexually transmitted diseases can't be transmitted from woman to woman. Vaginal secretions may carry bacteria and viruses—including HIV—so unless you're absolutely certain that your partner has no sexually transmitted infection, you must practice safer sex. Use a dental dam, Glide dams, a condom, or rubber glove that has been cut open or a piece of plastic wrap to cover her vulva, vagina, and anus during oral sex. Place a drop of water-based lubricant on the side that will be touching your partner to increase her pleasure. Safer sex practices are particularly important if you practice oral sex while your partner is having her period.

Chapter 10
Delicacy #5: Anal Sex

Though most are embarrassed to talk about it and few will even admit that they indulge in anal pleasure, 20 percent of women have experienced anal intercourse, according to the National Health and Social Life Survey. Often a woman's sexual partner will ask to engage in anal sex. But women, too, have voiced a curiosity about and interest in experiencing anal stimulation. In some cultures, anal intercourse is an accepted way for a woman to maintain her "virginity" until marriage while still providing pleasure to her partner (and sometimes herself as well). Other women elect anal intercourse because they can indulge without worrying about the risk of pregnancy.

Of all the sexual practices, anal sex seems to be the most misunderstood. Myths and misconceptions abound. The following concerns are common among women:

Anal sex is painful. Anal sex play does not have to be painful. If you learn the proper techniques prior to experimenting, you may find it enjoyable. Some women and men can have orgasms from anal stimulation alone. Anal sex is not for everyone, however, and you may never find it enticing.

Inserting a finger or penis into your rectum can cause harm. If force is used to enter your anus, or if you're uncomfortable and not relaxed, injury can occur. However, it can be done safely by practicing proper technique.

The anus is dirty. As children we are taught early on that our backside is dirty; we must wipe carefully after going to the bathroom and then wash our hands thoroughly. Then again, you may have been told that the vagina is dirty, and we certainly are able to find wonderful ways to get pleasure out of vaginal stimulation.

The anus certainly has many bacteria, and daily cleaning is recommended. Because the bacteria here are different from the ones that naturally inhabit your vagina, to prevent vaginal infections you should not move a finger, penis, or toy from your anus to your vagina without washing it first.

Anal sex can give you AIDS. This is a common myth. If your partner is not infected with the HIV virus, anal sex won't give you AIDS. But if your partner is infected with HIV, the risk of transmitting the virus is higher during anal sex than during other sexual activities. It is advisable to use a condom during anal intercourse if you are not sure of his status.

I feel humiliated and degraded when I have anal intercourse. If you don't find anal sex appealing, then you shouldn't do it. You should never allow someone to force you to do something that you do not want to do. Remember, you are in control of what you do sexually.

Only homosexuals practice anal intercourse. Maybe my partner is gay. Many people mistakenly consider anal sex a purely homosexual act, but the desire for anal sex is unrelated to one's sexual identity. The truth is that heterosexual couples also participate in and enjoy anal sex play. It is simply another option for sexual gratification.

Anal sex is an unnatural act. You get to decide what feels natural to you. Since ancient times, anal sex has been an accepted practice in many cultures.

Anatomy of the Anus

To understand the ins and outs of anal sex play, you need to understand the anatomy of the anus and rectum.

If you spread the buttocks, you will notice the opening to the anus. The skin surrounding the opening is darker in color and contains hair and sweat- and oil-secreting glands. Beyond that opening is the anus itself, a tube that is 1½ inches long. It has no hair or glands, nor does it produce any secretions or lubrication, but the anus and the surrounding skin contain many nerve endings and are therefore very sensitive to touch and stretching.

The anus is surrounded by two rings of muscle, the external and internal *sphincters*. These sphincters hold the "tube" closed until you are ready to release waste. You have control of your external sphincter muscles—you can tighten and release them—but the internal sphincter muscles aren't under your control (involuntary) and will tighten automatically whenever something is pushed into your anus. Though it appears small and tight, the anus is capable of stretching enough to accommodate any sized penis.

At the top of the anus is the rectum, the lower part of the large intestine. As you go from the anus to the rectum, the rectum takes a sharp curve forward, in the direction of your stomach. The rectum then continues for another 5 inches and makes several turns. The rectum contains few nerves and is therefore much less sensitive than the anus, but some people enjoy the feeling of "fullness" that's created when an object is placed in the rectum. *Be careful: The tissue of the rectum is delicate and easily damaged by sharp objects.*

The prostate and the vagina lie in front of the rectum and can be stimulated through the thin anterior wall of the rectum.

Anal Sex Techniques

Analingus

Commonly known as "rimming," *analingus* is the stimulation of the anus with the mouth. Some men love the sensation of a warm wet tongue against their rectums; others absolutely hate the thought. Just ask before deciding to surprise him with your newfound knowledge.

Prior to analingus, it is important to clean the area around the anus with soap and water, so sharing a bath or shower is a great prelude to anal play. The easiest position for rimming is with your partner lying on his back with his knees bent. Placing a pillow under his buttocks will make access to his anus easier. Or you can have him pull his knees back toward his chest to bring his anus closer to you. First kiss and lick along his buttocks, moving closer and closer to his anus. Use your tongue to stimulate the opening to the anus and surrounding area. If you have a very strong tongue, you may be able to insert it a short distance into the anus.

As a doctor, I must also remind you about the possible dangers of this activity. Bacteria, parasites, hepatitis viruses, and sexually transmitted diseases can be picked up during analingus. *To be safe, you might want to use a dental dam or a piece of thin plastic wrap over the anus.*

Manual Anal Play

You can create many sensations using your fingers in and around the anus. Before you begin your exploration, you must be sure to cut your fingernails very short and smooth any ragged edges. Those French tips can cause a lot of damage to the walls of the anus and rectum. You can also use gloves, a condom, or a finger cot over your finger and nails to protect the anus from damage. The rectum and anus do not produce their own lubrication, so have lots of water-based lubricant available.

He should lie on his back with his knees bent and his legs open, while you kneel between his legs. Apply a generous amount of lubricant to the outside of the anus and on your middle finger. Gently stroke and massage the opening of his anus. If he becomes aroused and wants to go further, lightly press the anal opening with the pad of your finger. If you notice him tightening up, don't force your way inside. Maintain the same pressure until you notice the tightening loosen. Then it is safe to push your finger in a little further, entering with your hand palm up so that the finger points toward the stomach as it enters, following the natural course of the anus and rectum.

Go slowly. You will most likely notice a definite tightening of the anus as you push your finger further in—the anal spincters at work. Wait for a minute until those muscles relax: Massage or lick his scrotum, penis, and inner thighs while you wait. When you feel the tightening loosen, insert your finger further into the rectum. Another way to enter the anus is to have your partner push his bottom toward you while you keep your finger stationary. You might also ask him to bear down (as if having a bowel movement) to make the initial insertion easier.

When your finger is in as far as it can reach, begin a slow massage of the front wall of the rectum. You will notice a small bulge. That's the prostate gland, and stroking it can provide some men with indescribable pleasure. Just below the prostate you may feel a small soft dimple, which some men find as sensitive as the prostate—if not more so. To massage these areas, use the same motion that you would use if you were beckoning someone to "come here." You can intensify his experience by moving the finger in and out or in circles, or by vibrating the finger rapidly from side to side. Be sure to use lots of lubricant and replenish frequently to avoid injuring the delicate tissue. While stimulating his prostate, keep your other hand and mouth busy, too, by pleasuring his scrotum, perineum, penis. The combination of sensations can be delightful.

Some women also enjoy manual stimulation of their anus and rectum. If you want to try it, have your partner follow the instructions given above. He may be able to stimulate the sensitive anterior wall of the vagina (G-spot) through your rectum by firm strokes of the front wall of your rectum.

Anal Intercourse

Before you embark on anal intercourse, first and foremost make sure that you and your partner both want this experience. If one of you is reluctant to participate, it will be hard for you to relax, your muscles are more likely to remain tense, and the experience won't be a positive one. So have a

A Common Concern

There are no feces in the anus, and the lower rectum is usually free of waste, but sometimes a small amount may remain. If you're concerned about the possibility of running into waste, wear a glove. You can also ask your partner to use an enema to clean the lower rectum prior to anal sex.

frank discussion with your partner about your concerns, and practice with other anal techniques before you progress to intercourse. Spend a little time with manual stimulation of the anus to get your body used to the sensations. Sometimes practicing with a small dildo is also helpful in training the muscles of the anus to relax.

When you're ready to begin, you will need lots of lubricant—water-based if you are using a condom. (If you are in any way unsure about the health status of your partner, you should be using one. The HIV virus may be transmitted through small tears or abrasions in the rectum during intercourse, as can herpes, warts, human papilloma virus, syphilis, gonorrhea, and chlamydia.) The thicker lubricants, such as "probe" or "K-Y Jelly," are good for anal intercourse, but avoid the use of spermicidal jelly (like the ones you use with your diaphragm) as a lubricant. Nonoxynol-9, the most common spermicide, has been shown to irritate the tissue of the rectum.

Discard the condom and use a different one if you plan to follow anal intercourse with vaginal intercourse.

There are many positions that can be used for anal intercourse. Experiment and find the one that is most comfortable for you. The most common positions include:

> 🔖 You lie on your side while he lies behind you, spoon fashion, and enters from the rear.

֍ He kneels behind you while you are on your hands and knees. This position gives you the deepest penetration.

֍ He lies on his back while you squat, facing him, and lower your bottom onto his penis. This position gives you more control of how deep the penis is allowed to go.

֍ You lie on your back with your hips elevated on pillows and your knees pulled back. He enters from above.

֍ You lie on your stomach and he lies on top.

Begin by applying a generous amount of lubricant at the opening to your rectum and along the shaft and head of his penis. He should lubricate his fingers and gently massage the opening to your anus until you become more aroused and he can enter your anus with his finger, spreading lubricant higher into your anus.

Communication is very important here. You shouldn't feel rushed or in pain. If anything hurts, tell your partner. Stop what you are doing, wait, and start again later if you wish. If you are enjoying what he is doing, share that with him as well. It will help him know how to proceed.

Once you've loosened up, he should place the penis at the entrance to your anus and apply light pressure, then slowly slide the penis a little further into the anus. It sometimes helps if you slide your anus toward his penis and bear down. The internal sphincter muscles will tighten, resisting the entry of the penis somewhat and making you feel as though you need to have a bowel movement. This is a normal reaction and will pass. *Never force the penis into the anus or rectum, or you may cause tears or cracks in the delicate tissue.*

Tell him to keep the penis still until your muscles relax and you're ready to proceed with deeper penetration. Then he can slowly slide the penis deeper into the rectum a little at a time. Once inside, the two of you can move together to find the stroke and rhythm that work best for both of you. Be creative. If at any time you feel that the anus is becoming dry, add more lubrication. Semen is not irritating to the anus or rectum.

Advanced Anal Sex Play

If you find that anal sex play is a real turn-on, try adding toys to your routine. You might want to use a butt plug—a dildo with a flared base so the toy cannot get lost in the rectum. Vibrators can also be used to stimulate the outside of the anus.

Keeping It Safe

Using a condom during anal sex will protect you from most sexually transmitted infections. The human papilloma virus may be transmitted even with a condom, and some types may cause anal cancer. Many doctors do not check the anus routinely, so be sure to let your doctor know that you indulge in anal intercourse. Anal inspection, culture, and a rectal pap smear (similar to the cervical pap smear) may be recommended.

Chapter 11
Delicacy #6: Intercourse

Women are encouraged to learn life skills like how to sew, bake, type, and even change the tires on their car. But they aren't taught how to have pleasurable intercourse. In my practice, I have seen more than a few women who were unable to consummate their marriages because of lack of knowledge regarding intercourse.

Our parents' birds-and-bees talk—if we got one—usually just covered the basics. If we think beyond that, we usually assume that nature will take its course and somehow we will just know what to do when the time arrives to have intercourse. Many of us also assume that our male partner will know what to do. But his birds-and-bees talk was probably as basic as yours, and the locker-room talk may have left him even less informed. Even being "experienced" doesn't help much if the experiences weren't good ones.

You might think, "How can it be at all complicated to put a penis inside a vagina?" Well, for the most part, it isn't. Unfortunately, once it's in, people often don't know what to do next. For some, intercourse is a very mechanical act. The woman lies there while the man thrusts his penis back and forth until he reaches orgasm. The average man can climax in 3 minutes while the average woman needs at least 12–15 minutes, so you can see right there that rudimentary sex isn't necessarily going to be pleasing to both of you. He's more likely to be satisfied than you are.

If all of this sounds grim, it shouldn't. First off, the facts above should help you see that if your sexual experiences haven't been great, there's a reason—and it isn't necessarily your fault. Great lovemaking is a learned skill. The learning process can be loads of fun, and in the end, you'll get much more pleasure from the experience.

Starting Points

Knowledge of your body and how it responds as well as good communication with your partner are key to great vaginal intercourse. Before jumping into the sack, you need to ask yourself a few questions.

"Do I need contraception?"

Unlike other delicacies, unprotected vaginal intercourse can lead to pregnancy; if you don't want a baby, you need to be thoroughly protected. The time to think about contraception is before you get into bed—even before you begin to get passionate. Once the two of you are in the throes of passion, it may be difficult to think rationally, and you certainly won't want to interrupt your necking and petting to run out to the corner drugstore. I've received hundreds of panicked calls from women who only realized the ramifications of unprotected intercourse after it was over, so be prepared.

"Do I need protection against sexually transmitted infections?"

If you're with a new partner whose sexual history is unfamiliar to you, you'll want to be protected from sexually transmitted infections (STIs). Again, the time to discuss protection against STIs is before you get in bed. Just taking his word that he doesn't have any infections is not enough. Unfortunately, you may not get the truth when things have begun to heat up.

Besides, he may be unaware that he has an infection. Until you can be certain that he is safe, don't take chances. Life is too short.

"Am I emotionally prepared to deal with the aftermath of intercourse?"

Sex is considered recreation by some—no more serious than a vigorous game of tennis. However, engaging in sexual intercourse can have serious, sometimes unexpected, emotional consequences for women. In my practice I have counseled many women who found themselves "stuck like glue" to men after having intercourse. One woman told me that she will never have casual sex again because she woke up "in love" with a man after their first date ended with "fantastic sex."

Women most commonly engage in intercourse because of feelings of love or affection; men don't necessarily enter into sexual relationships with the same emotional investment. Decide beforehand exactly what this sexual encounter means to you. Ask yourself why you want to sleep with him. Have you established a relationship and it seems to be the right time? Do you think it will make him fall in love with you? Do you just think he's gorgeous and want to get next to that body? Are you looking for comfort or an emotional connection? Will you be devastated if he doesn't call you in the morning—or the next day? Are you afraid he'll stray if you don't have sex with him?

You can't make a man fall in love with you through intercourse. If the sex is good, he may "lust" after you, but lust does not equal love. You can enjoy a happy-go-lucky sexual romp if that's what you're looking for. If you're with someone who's emotionally compatible with you, the encounter can be amazingly comforting. Make sure you aren't convincing yourself that mutual affection exists to justify intercourse. Don't be pressured into intercourse for any reason. Make a well-thought-out, mature, personal decision.

Sexual Moves

In Victorian times women were told not to move at all during intercourse; the action was up to the man. Unfortunately, that historic holdover still makes some women feel that "ladies" don't move too much when they're having sex. Really, sex is like a dance between two partners who alternate the lead role, each contributing to the final masterpiece. You should feel free to move.

Chances are good that even if you lie as still as a piece of petrified driftwood, your partner will still get his, but the likelihood that you'll have an orgasm will be much less. Fortunately, there are movements you can do that will greatly increase the pleasure for both of you.

Practice the moves below while standing, and when you get in bed, practice the moves while lying on your back and then on your stomach.

Pelvic Tilt

Stand with your feet shoulder-width apart, knees slightly bent, stomach in, shoulders back, and head straight. (Each standing move will begin with this basic standing position.) Push your pelvis forward by contracting your buttock muscles. Keep your feet flat and isolate your pelvis so your torso doesn't move. Release by relaxing your buttock muscles and returning to the basic stance. Repeat.

When lying on your back, repeat the movements first with your knees bent and then with the knees and legs straight and with your legs apart. Also practice the tilt while lying on your stomach and while kneeling on your knees.

Some women never venture past the tilt. To increase the chance that your hot spot will be stroked during intercourse, you should study and practice the moves that follow.

Swaying Hips

Standing, move your right hip out to the side by putting your weight onto your left leg, then shift the hips to the left, putting the weight onto your right leg. Don't move your torso, just your hips. As you shift the weight onto one leg, that knee may straighten slightly, but don't let it stiffen or lock, or your movements will be jerky. All movement should be smooth and continuous. Now sway your hips while lying on your back, stomach, and knees.

Twisting Hips

This is an advanced variation of the pelvic tilt. From the basic standing position, isolate the right and left buttock, or gluteal, muscles. Swivel your right hip forward by contracting the right gluteal muscles as you move the hip. Return to center and then contract the left gluteal muscle as you move the left hip forward. Return to center and repeat the steps. Your movements should be smooth as you twist your hips from side to side. Practice while lying on your back, stomach, and while kneeling. You can also choose to isolate one side to the exclusion of the other side if you wish.

With this move you and your partner will enjoy interesting sensations while you are on top kneeling on your knees. It helps when you want to move the penis to different areas inside the vagina during intercourse, or if your hot spot is in an area that is difficult to reach with the straight pelvic tilt.

The Stair-Climbing Move

From the standing position, move your right hip straight up (toward your head), straightening your right knee slightly as your right heel lifts from the floor. Lower your foot and hip, and return to starting position. Repeat with the left hip and continue, alternating in smooth and flowing movements. This movement is especially nice when you are lying on top with the penis deep inside.

Hip Circles

Assume the basic standing position. Begin by making a square with your hips. Push your hips forward, move your hips to your right, move your hips straight back, then to your left, then forward, and finally back to the center. You have now completed a square. The next step is to round out the corners.

Imagine there is a circle on the floor and you are standing in the center of the circle. Now trace the circle with your hips. Your hips should move smoothly around the circle: forward, right, back, left, forward. Your torso and feet should not move.

Vary the size of the circles from large to very small and then speed up from slow to fast. Vary the direction by moving clockwise and counterclockwise. You can drive him wild by changing direction and speed at the same time.

This move can be varied and expanded to achieve incredible sensations and is the best movement for stimulating the clitoris. You can maximize stimulation of the clitoris by lying on top or by kneeling with your torso leaning forward over your lover. As you circle, the clitoris is rubbed alternately against his pubic bone and the base of his penis. The top of the penis is moved about the top and walls of the vagina, stimulating many areas of the vagina.

Up-and-Down Hip Circles

Stand with your legs slightly parted and your knees straight. Move your pelvis straight back using your lower back muscles. Now lower your pelvis by bending your knees slightly. With your knees still bent, contract your buttocks and thrust your pelvis straight forward. Now raise your pelvis by straightening your knees. Repeat until the movements are fluid and smooth. It may help to imagine that your pelvis is in the center of a circle that is slicing your body into left and right halves. Trace the circle with your pelvis. As you push your pelvis back and down, you are tracing one half, and as you continue the movement forward and up, you are tracing the other half of the circle. You can reverse the direction of the circle by moving your pelvis forward, down, back, and up. Once mastered, it will give you years of pleasure while sitting on top of your lover.

Side-to-Side Figure Eight

This is an advanced move and must be practiced before using it during intercourse. Once you get good at it though, you will love it and so will he! Assume the basic standing position. Imagine the number 8 on the floor. Your body is at the center of the 8 with your right foot in one circle and your left foot in the other circle. Now trace the 8 with your hips. Push your right hip forward, then to the right side, then back, then center. Your left hip then moves forward, to the left, back, forward, and center. Repeat until your moves are fluid and sensual. Do not move your feet or torso during the hip moves. Vary the size of the 8 and the speed that you trace it. This move is fabulous when he is sitting in a chair and you are straddling him or while you're in the missionary position.

Front-to-Back Figure Eight

This move is the same as the one above except that the 8 is front to back. Stand in the middle of an imaginary figure 8. One circle is in front of you and one is behind you. Trace the 8 with your hips. Move your left hip to the left, forward, to the right, back, center, then left, back, right, forward, and center. Repeat the steps and make sure your moves are smooth and fluid.

Hip Vibration Moves

These small, subtle, and very rapid moves are the most advanced and require lots of practice. Perfect them, and you are worth your weight in gold.

Lie on your back with your knees slightly bent. Contract your buttock muscles, lifting your hips. Now relax your butt and lower your hips. Repeat this move faster and faster. As you increase the speed, the movements become smaller until only your buttock muscles are making small rapid contractions. It will feel as if your pelvis is vibrating. Try contracting your pelvic floor muscles at the same time.

You can vary this vibration move by moving your hips rapidly from side to side. Again, only your alternating buttock muscles are contracting. These moves are great if the penis remains stationary and deep inside the vagina. Women who love stimulation of the upper vagina and cervix will adore this move.

Positions

If you've ever read the Kama Sutra or seen one of the ancient Chinese sex guides, you know that people have been experimenting with new sexual positions for hundreds of years. In fact, hundreds of sexual positions have been described over the centuries. Some of them could only be done by a pair of double-jointed acrobats, but there are still certainly many others that the average person can enjoy.

Basically, most sexual postures are based on one of six basic position types: woman on top, man on top, rear entry, side to side, sitting, and standing. You can try the variations that fall under one of the categories, or you can change positions several times during an episode of intercourse. However, changing positions too frequently can be distracting and disruptive to the flow of lovemaking. Learn how to change from one position to the next without withdrawing the penis for a real erotic experience. Experiment and find the positions that work best for you and your partner. Remember to enjoy plenty of foreplay before you get into any position. Vary the speed of your movements as well as the angle and depth of penetration of his penis for sensational sex.

Woman-on-Top Positions

Some women shy away from the woman-on-top positions because they're afraid that their partner will view them as too assertive or aggressive. The truth is that most men enjoy these positions because they don't have to work as hard and they love being able to see their lover's face and body. Besides, variety is exciting, and these positions allow more freedom of movement for the woman. You can move your pelvis such that you control the depth of penetration and speed of thrusting as well as increase the stimulation of your clitoris or G-spot during intercourse. Some women find that they can only orgasm in the woman-on-top positions. Here are some variations:

> Have your partner lie flat on his back while you straddle his pelvis with your knees. When you're both ready, place the penis at the opening of your vagina and slowly lower your pelvis down onto it. Start with shallow penetration and, as you become more comfortable, lower your body further until you are in a sitting position. Penetration is quite deep in this position. Encourage him to use his hands to touch and stimulate your clitoris and breasts to further your enjoyment. Making eye contact with your partner increases the intimacy between you.

≫ You can increase penile stimulation of the clitoris by leaning your upper body forward and lowering yourself onto your partner's chest. As you raise your pelvis up, push backward against his penis, stroking your clitoris as you come up. As you stroke down, move your pelvis forward. Your motions are more like back-and-forth rocking than like thrusting movements. In the beginning, ask your partner to remain still, but as you get more stimulated, he should join you in the rocking movements. You can reverse this movement by moving your pelvis down and back against the penis on the downstroke, sliding your clitoris against the penis. Your pelvis then moves forward and up on the upstroke.

≫ With your partner lying flat on his back, kneel over him, and lower yourself onto his penis. Once it's fully inserted, straighten your legs behind you and lie flat with your full weight on top of your partner. Total body contact increases intimacy and will encourage mutual kissing and caressing. In this position there's shallower penile penetration, but your clitoris will be stimulated more during thrusting. Your partner will also notice more friction against his penis. Add to your mutual enjoyment by contracting your PC (pubococcygeus) muscles and use sexual moves to force the penis against your clitoris and other sensitive spots. For a different sensation your partner can wrap his legs around the outside of your legs, or you can spread your legs on either side of his closed and outstretched legs.

≫ Straddle your partner's pelvis with your knees. After the penis is fully inserted, lean back and balance yourself with your hands as you begin to move together. The anterior wall of your vagina is stroked and massaged by his penis creating a new sensation, and he can add to your pleasure by manually stimulating your clitoris or placing a vibrator there. The vibrations will spread to the base of his penis, giving you both a new erotic experience. Some men, however, will find the backward pressure on their penis to be uncomfortable, especially if their erection tends to angle more toward their abdomen.

Woman on Top—Legs Straight

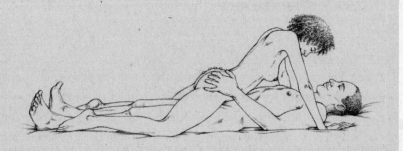

Woman on Top—Legs Bent

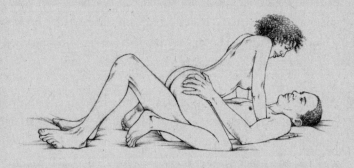

Woman on Top—Cradling

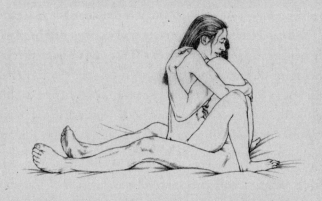

⟩ You can also get into woman-on-top positions by beginning with the man on top and—being careful to keep him inside you—roll over together.

Man-on-Top Positions

The best known man-on-top position is the *missionary position,* and most man-on-top positions are just variations. This position allows the man to be in control of the thrusting and do most of the "work." This may be unfair, but it's worth it, because men get more stimulation in these positions and may find it easier to reach orgasm. Meanwhile, the woman can lie back and enjoy the feeling of being "made love to." But she doesn't have to be passive and will increase her enjoyment by actively participating in the dance.

In the basic missionary position, you lie on your back with your knees slightly bent and legs parted. He lies on top and supports his body weight with his elbows and arms. His legs are between yours, allowing deep penetration of your vagina. You can try variations from there.

⟩ Assume the missionary position. When the penis is fully inserted, lower and close your legs. He can keep his legs straight, straddle either side of your legs, or place one leg in between your legs and the other on the outside of your legs. Each will give a different sensation. Penetration isn't deep, but you'll experience greater stimulation of your clitoris as the penis passes over your vulva on the way to your vagina. And there's more friction on the penis, creating a different pleasurable sensation for your partner.

You can increase the stimulation of your clitoris by placing a firm pillow under your buttocks. This thrusts your pelvis further forward, increasing the exposure of your clitoris to his penis. For an entirely different sensation, your partner can rotate his body 45 degrees across your body. This will cause the penis to stroke the side of your vagina rather than the anterior or posterior walls.

⟩ From the missionary position, pull your knees back toward your chest. The further back you can pull your knees, the deeper the

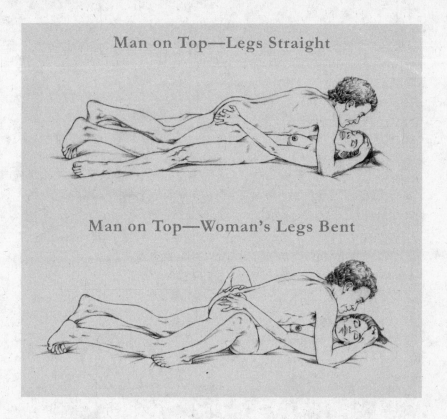

Man on Top—Legs Straight

Man on Top—Woman's Legs Bent

penetration. If you are flexible enough, try putting your feet on his shoulders or even around his neck. The clitoris receives no attention, but the anterior wall of the vagina and cervix are well stimulated. This position is great for women who love very deep penetration and thrusting, but because the penetration is so deep, some women will find this position uncomfortable, especially during ovulation and just before the menses.

Assume the missionary position, and when the penis is inserted, wrap your legs around his thighs. Your partner should then move his pelvis forward a couple of inches so that his pelvis is closer to your navel than to your pelvis. The base of his penis is now pressed against your mons, the top of your labia majora, and the shaft of your clitoris, and the head of his penis is in your vagina. You're supporting the full weight of his body. (This po-

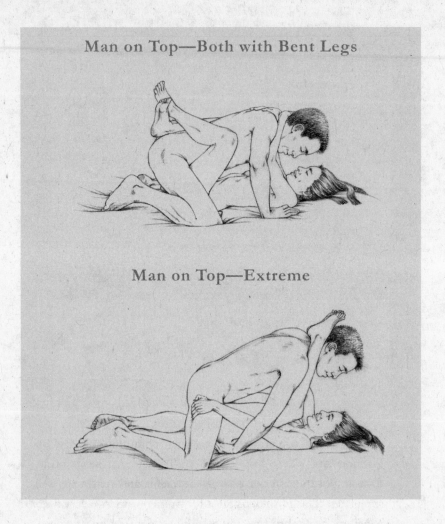

Man on Top—Both with Bent Legs

Man on Top—Extreme

sition may not work well if he is much heavier than you or if you are much shorter than he is, but it is worth a try.) The movement is not a thrusting but rather a back-and-forth rocking movement in which both partners do half the work. You begin the upward stroke, moving your pelvis up and forward. The penis strokes the clitoris as it is pushed further into the vagina. Your partner then takes over during the downward stroke, moving his pelvis down and pushing your pelvis down and backward. You can increase the pressure against your clitoris by pressing it against the base of his penis as he forces your pelvis down. Rock back and forth together at a steady, comfortable pace. If it all sounds complicated, that's because it is—but it is well worth the effort and practice to get it right. This position was described and coined the *coital alignment* technique by Edward W. Eichel, a sex therapist.

▧ Lie flat on your back and slide your buttocks to the edge of the bed and hang your legs over. Your partner stands or kneels in front of you, depending on the height of the bed, and enters your vagina. Clitoral stimulation is increased if he leans his body over your body, pressing the shaft of his penis against your vulva. Vaginal penetration can be increased if you wrap your legs around his waist or if he lifts your pelvis with his hands as he thrusts.

Rear-Entry Positions

Some people hate rear-entry positions, often complaining that they are primitive and "animalistic" because most animals copulate this way. This is exactly the reason that others find these positions so enticing. These positions are also good for stroking your G-spot.

▧ Kneel on your hands and knees. Your partner kneels upright behind you and enters your vagina from the rear. Penetration is deep, and the anterior wall of the vagina is stroked. Your movements are limited in this position, and your partner does most of the thrusting. His hands are free to stimulate your clitoris, breasts, and buttocks, but you are unable to touch him. Some of the intimacy is lost because you cannot see each other.

▧ You can increase the stimulation of your clitoris by lowering your torso and placing your weight on your elbows. Your pelvis is pushed backward and upward, increasing the contact between the shaft of his penis and your clitoris. You may find that you get somewhat dizzy if this position is held for a prolonged period of time.

Rear-Entry—Upright on Knees

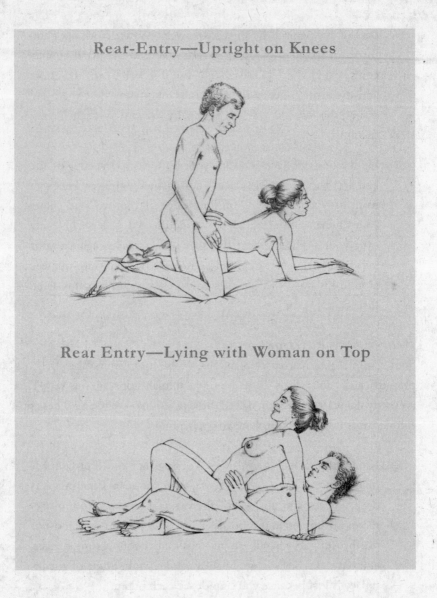

Rear Entry—Lying with Woman on Top

⚘ Stand at the side of the bed and lean over, putting your weight on your elbows. Your partner stands behind you and enters from the rear.

⚘ From there you can lie flat on your stomach and let your partner lie on top of you with his legs straight or straddling your legs.

The penis enters from the rear. The penetration is shallow but can be increased by placing a pillow under your pelvis, elevating it. Use your buttock muscles to squeeze his penis as he thrusts.

Your partner lies on his back. You turn your back to him and straddle his pelvis, lowering yourself onto his penis. Some people don't like having their back to their partners; it decreases intimacy. Others find it easier to fantasize and self-stimulate in this position.

Side-to-Side Positions

Side-to-side positions are good when the two of you are tired and want to have slow, relaxed intercourse. With both of you lying on your side facing

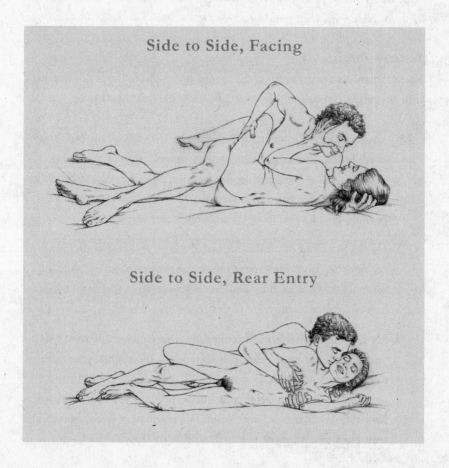

Side to Side, Facing

Side to Side, Rear Entry

each other, you lift your top leg so that he can insert his penis into your vagina. The higher you lift, the deeper the penetration can be and the more he can stimulate your clitoris with his hand. Keeping your legs straight and closed will decrease the depth of penetration but increase the stimulation of your clitoris. You are both limited in your movements, but you each have one hand free to stroke and massage each other as you gaze into each other's eyes.

You can also lie on your side and have him lie on his side behind you so he can enter from the rear. You may have to lean forward a little to allow penetration. Your bodies should then fit together like two spoons—not surprisingly, this is known as the *spoon position*. This position is very sensual because you have total body contact and his top hand is free to caress your body or stroke your clitoris. Alternatively, you are free to stroke your clitoris yourself with your hand or a sex toy.

Sitting Positions

These positions are great for a change of pace. They all put his face near your breasts, so he can nibble your nipples while he's inside you.

- Your partner sits in an armless chair or on the edge of the bed. You sit on his lap, lowering your vagina down and onto his penis much as you would in a woman-on-top position. You're in control of the depth of penetration and have freedom to move your pelvis. This position enables you to kiss, touch, and caress each other.

- He sits in a chair or on the edge of the bed, and you sit on his lap facing away from him. Your movement is not hindered, but the intimacy is decreased as you face away from your partner. His hands are free to massage your breasts and clitoris.

- He lies flat on his back. Facing him, you straddle his pelvis on your knees. After the penis is inserted into the vagina, your partner should pull his body up to the sitting position and you should straighten your legs, bend your knees, or wrap your legs around his back. You can hold each other in a sensual caress, or you can lean back and support yourself with your hands. Movement is

limited for both of you, but you can contract your pubococcygeus (PC) muscles for internal stimulation of the penis and to
increase your own sensations.

Standing Positions

These positions work well if you and your partner are close to the same
height. If one is much taller than the other, more advanced acrobatics are
required.

You and your partner stand facing each other. One of you places your
back against a wall. You spread your legs and guide the penis into your
vagina. Penetration is shallow, but the clitoris is stimulated as the penis enters the vagina. If you close your legs, the stimulation of the clitoris is very
intense. You can increase the depth of penetration if your partner supports your buttocks while you wrap your legs around his pelvis and lean
with your back against the wall.

For a change, have your partner enter you from the rear while standing.
You may need to lean your torso forward to effect penetration.

Lubrication

Your vagina naturally lubricates when you become sexually aroused.
Sometimes, however, the amount of lubrication that you produce is not
enough for intercourse. Women need more stimulation than men to prepare for intercourse, and the amount of stimulation needed increases as
we age. Lubrication may be decreased by birth control pills, pregnancy,
childbirth, breast feeding, vaginal infections, menopause, douching, and
some medications. You may also notice that your vaginal secretions are
lighter during some parts of your menstrual cycle, while under stress, and
sometimes for no reason at all.

Water-based lubricants are available to supplement your natural vaginal
lubrication. Many women have voiced reluctance to using lubricants because they don't want to be seen as "dried up" or "frigid." Some have told
me that lubricants are too "artificial." Even if your natural lubrication is
more than adequate, lubricants can be fun and may add new sensations to
your lovemaking. Introduce them during foreplay. Invite your partner to

help choose the lubricant of the evening. Smell, taste, and compare the consistency of several lubricants and choose the one that you both like best. Some people like the watery, thin lubricants, while others like the thicker or viscous variety. It's all a matter of personal taste. You can purchase flavored lubricant, but don't expect "pineapple" to taste like it was just flown in from Hawaii. Do not use flavored lubricants inside the vagina; they may cause vaginal infections.

There are many brands of lubricants. All contain purified water and inert plastics, and most contain a preservative. Some can be purchased from your local pharmacy, and others must be purchased from an adult shop or ordered from an adult specialty catalog or over the Internet. Be sure to order a water-based lubricant if you will be using a latex condom; an oil-based lubricant can damage condoms. If you become irritated after using a lubricant, do not continue to use it. Check the ingredients, and try another brand with different ingredients. For instance, some women get frequent yeast infections with lubricants containing glycerin but may do well with one containing silicone. Petroleum jelly (Vasoline), a commonly used lubricant, is oil based, difficult to remove, and may increase your risk of vaginal infection.

You and your partner should experiment and figure out how much lubricant is just right. Using too much can decrease the friction and sensations that you feel during intercourse.

I took a field trip to two New York shops for a product test. There are many lubricants out there that I didn't test, and of course, I had my own favorites among the ones I tried. But you should try a few and make your own decision.

K-Y Jelly: The oldest lubricant used for intercourse, it can be purchased in your local pharmacy. It was not created specifically to be a sexual lubricant but rather to make insertion of medical devices and performance of medical exams easier. K-Y is thick and tends to dry out and become sticky during prolonged sex. It has a strong chemical taste.

K-Y Silk-e: Made by the manufacturers of K-Y Jelly, it is smooth, creamy, and odorless but has a strong taste. It contains vitamin E and can be used as a daily genital moisturizer if you have dryness of the vulva and vagina. It contains sorbitol, another sugar, so don't use it if you have frequent yeast infections.

K-Y Liquid: Also made by the manufacturers of K-Y Jelly, it is a thinner, clear, odorless lubricant. It has a strong taste and contains glycerin and sorbitol. Be careful if you are prone to frequent yeast infections. You can find it in your local pharmacy.

Astroglide: A slippery, clear lubricant, it is one of the most popular and one of the first lubricants made specifically for sex. You can find it in your local pharmacy. It does have lots of glycerin and may become sticky with prolonged sex, but you can remedy that by adding water to your genitals during sex. It is odorless but has a slight chemically sweet taste. It also comes in prefilled vaginal applicators under the brand name Silken Secret. The applicator makes insertion into the vagina easier and is especially great for postmenopausal women with vaginal dryness.

Venus: Smooth and silky in texture, because it's silicone based, it should not be used with silicone toys because it will bond with them, causing discomfort when you attempt to manipulate or remove the toy. It

Keeping It Safe

Intercourse can be mind-blowing, but it can also be dangerous if your partner has a sexually transmitted infection. Using a latex or polyurethane condom every time you have sex will decrease your risks. Use plenty of water-based lubricants to decrease the chances that the condom will break. A female condom protects as well as a male condom and gives you the control.

coats the skin so it lasts longer and is good for anal or vaginal intercourse. It is wonderful for menopausal women with dryness, especially those who are not on estrogen.

Bare: This lubricant comes in a cute bear-shaped container and has a lighter consistency than others. It contains a small amount of glycerin, is tasteless and odorless, and some women say that it feels more like natural vaginal secretions.

Probe: This contains glycerin and a natural preservative—grapefruit seed extract. It is long lasting and can be used for anal or vaginal intercourse. It has a slight chemically sweet taste. It's good even if you are allergic to chemical preservatives.

Sylk: Considered a "natural" lubricant, it contains only an extract of kiwi fruit vine and water with a minimal amount of preservative. It is wonderful for women with sensitive skin, but it doesn't taste very good.

Eros: A silicone-based, long-lasting lubricant, it is odorless and tasteless. The salespeople told me it can be used in the Jacuzzi, which let me know that it can be difficult to remove with a quick shower. It is good for anal or vaginal sex.

Maximus and For Play Cream: Thick, slippery lubricants that are considered to be two of the best for anal intercourse.

Liquid Silk: A smooth and creamy lubricant that stays wet longer and does not get sticky even with prolonged sex. It is white and creamy colored and looks a little like fresh semen. It contains no glycerin but has a strong taste. The feel is very natural.

Wet: A silicone-based lubricant, it is thicker and good for anal sex. It is colorless and odorless but has a strong taste.

Chapter 12

Sexual Enhancers

Just like anything you do over and over for years on end, sex can become predictable and routine. Fortunately, there are many easy and interesting ways for you to put some pizzazz back into your sex life. In this chapter, we'll talk about sexual enhancers and techniques for adding a little spark to your love life.

Fantasies

Sex is fantasy, friction, and frequency.
> —Michael A. Perelman, Ph.D.,
> Sex and Couples Therapist

One of the safest, most exciting pleasures you can add to your sexual repertoire is sexual fantasy. Fantasies are in fact a very normal form of sexual expression, and studies show that 95 percent of women fantasize at some time or other.

What Are Fantasies?

Your brain is your largest sex organ, and your mind is your body's most sensitive erogenous zone. You can look at fantasy as "mental masturbation." In fantasy, you create arousing scenarios in your mind, private thoughts that can provide excitement and pleasure. Fantasies may consist of fleeting sexy thoughts, or they may be extended dramas with a wide range of characters in elaborate imaginary scenes. They may be remembrances of a particularly pleasant past sexual experience or mental images of a sexual experience that you would like to try. But having a fantasy does not mean that you want to act it out. In fact, some of your most arousing fantasies may be about acts that you would never consider doing.

The brain is more powerful than we give it credit. Medical science has proven that, through thought alone, we can cause physical changes in our body. Studies show, for example, that your mind can decrease your blood pressure, strengthen your heart, and boost your immune system. A recent study by researchers at Johns Hopkins University showed that fantasies about pleasurable sexual activity can decrease your perception of pain. If this is the case, then it follows that you'd be able to use your mind—your fantasies—to get your love juices flowing. In fact, studies have also shown that women who fantasize have better sex and more orgasms. Fantasies can spice up your sex life, boosting your libido and your sexual pleasure.

Benefits of Fantasy

Fantasy is commonly used by sex therapists to treat problems of desire, arousal, and orgasm.

> *Desire:* An erotic fantasy can be a powerful private aphrodisiac. Creating pleasurable romantic or sexual images in your brain can boost your desire for sex. Thinking about a pleasurable sexual experience during nonsexual activities may help to get you in a sexy mood. Try thinking of your favorite fantasy hours before a planned sexual encounter. The anticipation that it creates will fan your flames of desire.

≫ *Arousal:* Fantasy helps to increase your arousal by focusing your mind on your lovemaking and on the sensations that you are experiencing. It can decrease distractions, like outside noise, which can interfere with your arousal. We have all had the experience of having our sexual buildup interrupted by lists of things to do and thoughts of problems at work or with the kids.

≫ *Orgasm:* Pleasurable erotic thoughts can intensify your physical sensations, and some women find it easier to orgasm while having a fantasy. Fantasy focuses your mind and in so doing may lessen your concern about your performance during sex and make your experience more enjoyable. A few women can even orgasm from fantasy alone.

≫ *Safe sex:* Fantasies are pure pleasure without any of the emotional or physical risks of actual intercourse: You can't get pregnant, contract an infection, get caught *en flagrant,* or even perform badly. In fantasy you can have a perfect body, perfect mate, and perfect sex.

≫ *Decreases boredom:* Fantasy can change routine sex into a new and exciting experience. If you have been having sex in the same place, in the same way, at the same time, with the same person, you can use fantasy for a total change of pace.

When to Fantasize

Fantasy and masturbation go hand in hand. Most women admit to using fantasy to guide them to orgasm during masturbation. In fact, studies show that women who used erotic fantasies to increase their pleasure while they masturbated also had more frequent orgasms when they had intercourse.

Fantasy during intercourse is a normal way to increase your enjoyment of sex, but many women feel guilty about it. Some fear that the use of fantasy means that something is missing in their relationship with their partner. If they are enjoying a fantasy during sex—especially if it involves someone other than their mate—then something must be wrong with them or with their partner, or at least with the sexual experience they are sharing. For others, fantasy during intercourse makes them feel as if they are deceiving their partners because it is not a shared activity.

More About Guilt

Studies show that about 24 percent of us feel guilty about our fantasies. Some women fear that fantasies are abnormal or immoral. Their guilt may be related to the fact that the sexual act they're fantasizing about seems inappropriate, or perhaps the person in the fantasy isn't someone that we "should" be having sex with—even fantasy sex. Our fantasies can under-

Women's Most Common Fantasies

- Reliving a past sexual experience
- Sex with your partner
- Sex with another man
- Sex with a woman
- Sex with more than one lover
- Sex in a new location
- Oral sex
- Forced sex
- A forbidden act
- Dominating a man

mine our image of ourselves as "good girls." Some religions teach that just *thinking* about a sexual act is the same as actually doing it—and doing it is forbidden—so fantasy leads to guilt and shame. Whatever the reasons for guilt, it can short-circuit any pleasurable feelings that you may have and can cause sexual dysfunction.

Allowing yourself to indulge in fantasy does not necessarily mean that you are dissatisfied with your partner, relationship, or sex life. They shouldn't interfere with your connection with your partner during intercourse. They are personal erotic thoughts to be enjoyed by you alone, and you don't have to share them unless you choose to.

Enjoy your fantasies. But fantasies can be a problem if:

- they are causing you to feel extreme guilt, fear, or shame;

- they are interfering with your ability to have a satisfying relationship with your partner;

- you feel a strong urge to act out a fantasy that will cause harm to yourself or someone else.

If any of these describe your experience, discuss it with your doctor or a therapist.

Sex Toys

My box of goodies arrived the week after Christmas, enclosed in a plain brown box. Such packages had become a common sighting during the holiday season, so my four-year-old grabbed the box from the mailman and charged down the hall toward me. "Mommy! Mommy! Look, another present! Open it! Open it!" he exclaimed. Noting the return address, I quickly told him that it wasn't a Christmas present but something for Mommy's work. He was disappointed, but he gave me the package and went off to play—and I set the box aside so that I could spirit it off to my office later. I was relieved. I still don't know how I would have explained the pink vibrator with the cute bunny ears had I not been home when the package arrived!

That's what buying sex toys has come to these days. Gone are the days when a woman had to wear a wig and other disguises to enter an adult store like the Pink Pussy Cat to purchase a toy. Today, safe, reputable, comfortable establishments can be found in every large city. And for women who find even the most discreet sex shop too much to handle, the Internet and mail-order catalogs offer a safe place to shop with the added benefit of anonymity. You can have even the most provocative toy delivered to your door in a plain cardboard box.

At one time, people thought of sex toys in terms of either the vibrator—the domain of the single woman who wasn't otherwise sexually active—or the handcuffs and studded leather gear used by people who were into the "kinky" stuff. Today, every woman can be open about having sex toys, whether she's a woman who uses her vibrator to help her enjoy her own private pleasures or a woman who has toys that she uses with her male or female lover. Everyone is discovering the variety of sensations and pleasure that toys can provide.

I often recommend sex toys to women in my practice because they are wonderful learning tools and great for "sexual rehabilitation." Sex toys can be helpful in teaching a woman how to reach orgasm. Those who are already orgasmic may find that with a vibrator they experience orgasms that are different and often much more intense than those produced during other sexual activity. Toys may be used by menopausal women to keep their vagina moist and healthy. They can relieve sexual tension and can be a lot of fun for just about anyone!

Vibrators

Vibrators were originally invented as a medical device sold only to doctors. Women who complained of a variety of symptoms, including fatigue, irritability, bloating, anxiety, headaches, erotic thoughts, vaginal secretions, or pelvic discomfort were thought to suffer from "hysteria." Doctors treated women with these conditions by using their fingers and oil to rub the woman's clitoris until she reached "hysterical paroxysm," medical jargon for what we know as orgasm. Some women needed only a few minutes of their doctor's assistance, but other women needed an hour or more. Even during the nineteenth century, doctors didn't have that much time to spend with a patient, and besides, even the most vigorous doctor's fingers would tire. So an electrical device was invented to assist the doctor in his treatment of his patients and improve upon his technique: The vibrator moved faster than the fingers and produced a stronger orgasm in less time, freeing the doctor to see more patients in the same amount of time without exhausting himself.

Initially used only in doctors' offices, vibrators became so popular that it wasn't long before smaller, portable ones were manufactured and sold directly to women for self-treatment of a number of ills. Even today, the most popular vibrator is marketed as a "massager" for sore muscles.

Electric Vibrators

Electric vibrators produce a strong vibration, and because they run on electric current, they won't die on you. They are more expensive than the battery-powered vibrators but are worth the investment because they last longer and produce more intense vibrations. Most are made by major home appliance manufacturers and are not marketed as sexual toys, but as muscle massagers. You can find them in the small-appliance section of pharmacies or department stores and, of course, shops that sell sex toys.

- Wand-type electric vibrators have a long handle topped by a round vibrating head. The most popular wand is the Hitachi Magic Wand. This large, somewhat noisy device has a soft head the size of a tennis ball and produces strong vibrations that spread out over a large area. The shape of this vibrator makes it easy to use in partner play.

- Coil-type electric vibrators run on an electromagnetic coil rather than a motor. They are shaped like small handheld electric mixers, with a vibrating head that's small so the vibrations are concentrated. Most come with attachments for stimulation of a variety of hot spots.

- The Wahl Swedish Massager straps onto the back of your hand and creates gentle vibrations as you touch yourself. It is more pleasurable for some women because it allows for direct skin-to-skin contact. Unfortunately, you may get a temporary numbness in your hand.

❧ The Eroscillator is a newer electric vibrator that looks like a cross between an electric toothbrush and a power drill. Don't be alarmed by the description, though. The Eroscillator claims to be more gentle to delicate tissues than the average vibrator. It provides safe but intense stimulation using side-to-side movement that produces intense orgasms. Be aware: You'll pay more for its concentrated effectiveness, and this brand is more difficult to find.

Battery-Powered Vibrators

Battery-powered vibrators come in hundreds of combinations of sizes, shapes, colors, and textures. Trying to decide which to purchase can be pretty daunting. I suggest that you try several of them!

❧ Smoothies are small, phallic-shaped, personal vibrators that look more like a very large tube of lipstick than a man's penis. Made of hard plastic, they come in a variety of colors and produce a vibration that is milder than that of an electric model and tends to be concentrated at the base of the Smoothie. If you are a beginner and want to start slowly, or if the idea of buying a "penis" is uncomfortable, try the Smoothie.

❧ The Pocket Rocket is the size of a small tube of lipstick and very portable. The vibrations are much stronger than you would expect from such a small toy. You can carry it in your purse for "unexpected emergencies."

❧ Penis look-alikes are made of a variety of materials, including hard rubber, vinyl, jelly rubber, silicone, and new materials designed to feel more like skin. They're shaped like the real thing (some even have veins and testicles), and some are curved at the tip to stimulate the G-spot. Batteries either go inside the vibrator or are attached to a power pack (the ones with the power pack produce stronger vibrations).

> Natural Contours vibrators were designed by a woman to fit the natural shape of the vulva. They are perfect for beginners.

> Dual-action vibes contain a penis look-alike that twirls and an attached "critter" (beaver, bear, rabbit, or kangaroo) that vibrates so that you can simultaneously stimulate your vagina and clitoris. They are great for women who like vaginal penetration but also need clitoral stimulation to reach orgasm.

> Eggs and Bullets are an excellent choice for someone new to vibrators. Designed to stimulate the clitoris, they're small and can be held in place with your hand or strapped to your body with a harness that can be worn during intercourse. Eggs and Bullets can be placed inside the vagina as well.

> Finger vibes are small vibrators powered by a watch battery and worn on your finger, allowing the intimacy of skin-to-skin contact. They can be used for masturbation or with a partner. The best of the bunch is the Fukuoku 9000.

Specialty Vibes

Peruse a sex toy catalog or Web site and you'll be surprised at the variety of vibrating sex toys they offer.

> Remote-controlled vibes allow you and your partner to have discreet sex play in public. They come in the form of panties or thongs with a remote control: You put on the undergarment and give the remote control to your partner. He or she operates from up to 20 feet away; so you never know when the "feeling" is going to hit you.

> Vibrating tongues—some with a liquid "saliva"—are designed to give you the sensation of cunnilingus.

> Auto vibrators can be plugged into the cigarette lighter of your automobile. (This may sound exciting, but please park before using one of these!)

ঌ Double vibrators can be shared with a partner or used in self-play to stimulate two orifices.

Using a Vibrator

Once you get your new toy, you have to figure out how to use it effectively. It's best to learn how to use the vibrator alone before sharing the fun with a partner.

Electric Vibes

If you've never used a vibrator before, you'll want to start slowly. Choose a time when you are not going to be disturbed and find a warm, comfortable, private place for your self-pleasuring. Along with your new vibrator, have some water-based lubricant on hand; it helps to protect your delicate tissues if you generously lubricate the vibrator and your vulva and vagina before you begin to play with your toy. Even if you feel wet, additional lubricant will increase your pleasure—and it's a good idea to prevent friction burns from the vibrator. For the most comfort, keep the lubricant at room temperature or warm it by wrapping the bottle or tube in a warm towel.

The easiest position for learning how to use a vibrator is probably lying on your back with your legs straight and slightly apart. Relax. Turn the vibrator on the low setting and move it—slowly and gently—across your mons and down your labia. If the vibrations feel too strong, or if you feel overwhelmed or uncomfortable, stop and cover your vulva with a small cloth to decrease the intensity of the sensations. As you become more comfortable with the feeling—and perhaps more aroused—you can expose more of your vulva and clitoris by bending your knees and opening your legs further. Continue to lightly move the vibrator along your mons and both labia and stroke the length of your clitoris. Some women find direct clitoral stimulation with a vibrator to be too intense; sliding the vibrator along the side of the clitoris is sometimes preferable. Concentrate on the sensations you're feeling, going slowly at first so that you can better determine which areas respond most pleasurably to the vibrator. You can increase the intensity of vibrations by applying more pressure, increasing the speed, or changing the way you move the vibrator along your body. Try to avoid leaving the vibrator in the same place for a prolonged period of time because the area may start to burn or become temporarily numb. If anything you're doing feels uncomfortable, stop and try again later.

Battery Vibes

If you've got a battery-operated vibrator, you can insert the top of it into warm water. Don't immerse it unless it's waterproof, and never immerse an electric toy in water. Then apply a generous amount of lubricant before use.

Begin as directed above. If you enjoy vaginal penetration, you can insert the smoothie or penis-shaped vibrator. Don't be surprised if you don't get much pleasure from vaginal thrusting with your vibrator. Most women find that the vibrator is much more effective and enjoyable when the clitoris is stimulated, either alone or simultaneously with the vagina. Most women do not orgasm from vaginal penetration alone.

Eggs and Bullets can be held against your clitoris with your hand or placed inside your panties for hands-free fun. Make sure you use lubrication.

Don't worry if you don't have an orgasm the first time you use your vibrator. Sometimes it can take weeks, and some women never reach the point of orgasm while using a vibrator.

Sharing Your Toys

More often these days, I find that couples are using toys to enhance their love lives, adding new dimensions to sex. Adding sex toys to your lovemaking does not mean that something is wrong or missing, or that the sex is not good enough. You use them to add to your repertoire of pleasuring techniques; they're not meant to replace your partner. No matter how realistic the dildo, it can hardly replace the warmth, love, and emotions of a partner. Sex toys can be used to add an element of fun and excitement to sex—and the pleasure they bring should be as thrilling for you as it is for your partner.

Vibrators can be used to provide both partners with simultaneous stimulation or you can alternate pleasuring each other. The Hitachi Magic Wand is particularly useful because of the long handle. Try placing the vibrating head between the two of you while in the sitting position. If you are having intercourse, place the vibrator against your clitoris while in a rear-entry or woman-on-top position. The vibrations will spread out and stimulate his penis as well. Small vibrators like eggs, bullets, and clit ticklers can be tucked between the two of you during intercourse or oral sex.

Keeping It Safe

- It is also important to practice safe sex when you're sharing your vibrator. Cover the vibrator with a condom and change condoms between uses. If the vibrator head is too large for a condom, you can cover it with a latex glove or cover your vulva with a dental dam or clear plastic wrap.

- Never, *ever* move a vibrator from the rectal area to the vaginal area. Cover the toy with a condom during anal stimulation, then remove it or change it before you stimulate the vaginal area.

- Always clean your vibrator between uses. You can use an antibacterial soap and water, alcohol and water, or commercial cleaners designed specifically for sex toys. After cleaning, rinse your toy well and air-dry if possible. Never put a vibrator into an airtight storage container while it's still moist.

- Avoid covering your vibrator with body powder containing talc. It may increase your risk of ovarian cancer.

- Never place a vibrator directly on a man's testicles; you might injure him.

- If you are allergic to latex, you may also react to toys made of jelly rubber. Stick to toys made of silicone or plastic.

- After prolonged use, battery-powered vibrators and battery packs may overheat. Do not lie on top of battery-powered vibrators for prolonged periods of time.

- Do not use a vibrator:

- on broken or inflamed skin,
- if you have an infection either inside your vagina or on your vulva,
- in or around your anus if you have hemorrhoids,
- on your legs if they are swollen or painful,
- that is designed for deep-heating massage. Massagers that deliver heat to sore aching muscles can severely burn the delicate tissues of your vulva, and you might not even notice until it is too late.

Dildos

A dildo is a penis-shaped toy that does not vibrate. Dildos can provide new pleasurable sensations when used during solo masturbation or with a partner. Dildos are not substitutes for a human penis but can enhance your sexual experience. They can be used for self-exploration in locating your hot spots—those that are slightly curved are especially useful if you are trying to locate your G-spot.

Dildos give you complete control of your sexual experience. You can determine when and how you are pleasured, how deep the penetration, how fast the thrusting, and even whether you are penetrated at all.

Buying a Dildo

You'll find dildos in the same shops, catalogs, and on-line sites that sell vibrators. If you can, visit a shop that specializes in sex toys so you can see and handle a variety of dildos firsthand. Dildos can be found in hundreds of colors, sizes, and shapes. You can find these sex toys made of rubber, jelly rubber, silicone, cyberskin, plastic, glass, stone, acrylic, aluminum—as well as age-old wood or leather. Dildos made of silicone are preferable because they are easy to clean and are durable. You'll find a variety of specialized dildos in your local sex shop.

Double dildos are long and have a head on each end. They're great for partner play because they can be used to penetrate you and your partner at the same time.

Strap-on dildos allow you to penetrate a partner. This role-reversal is a real turn-on for some women. You strap the dildo on with a harness made of leather or other fabrics and position it in front of your pubic bone like a penis.

A word of caution: If you are strapping on a dildo and penetrating the vagina or rectum of your partner, be aware that you can't easily determine when you meet resistance as you thrust, so it can be easy to damage your partner's delicate tissues. If this is a new experience for one or both of you, take it easy until you get used to this new play. Ask your partner always to let you know if he/she experiences any discomfort; be aware of his/her verbal and body cues at all times.

Using a Dildo

Dildos are made for vaginal penetration, but you might find they're wonderful when you use them to stimulate your clitoris as well. Be sure to use lots of water-based lubricants with your dildo even if you feel wet, and apply it regularly while you're playing because dildos will sometimes soak up lubrication during prolonged play. Begin by warming your dildo with warm water or a warm towel. Then slide the dildo around your mons and labia, stroking along the length of your clitoris and varying the pressure, speed, and direction of your strokes as you learn what feels most comfortable and sensual.

If you wish, you can slowly enter your vagina with the dildo. Limit yourself initially to the lower vagina only. Try starting at the mons and sliding all the way down the vulva and into the lower vagina. As you become more aroused, you can slide the dildo deeper into your vagina. Vary the depth of penetration, direction, and speed of your strokes.

Keeping It Safe

Clean your dildo before you use it the first time and after each use. If you are the only person using the dildo, clean it with antibacterial soap, rinse, and dry well. If you are sharing your dildo, cover it with a condom each time you use it. As with vibrators, condoms should also be used if you are using your dildo for stimulation of your anus and vagina or vulva. Be careful when you use dildos made of glass. Though they are marketed as "shatter-resistant," they can break.

Other Sex Toys

Ben-Wa Balls

An ancient toy, Ben-Wa Balls are two metal balls the size of cherries. To use them, you place them in your vagina then rock in a chair, roll your hips, dance, or jump up and down. As you move, the balls bump against each other and cause pleasing vibrations for some women. To increase the intensity of the sensation, you can contract your pubococcygeus (PC) muscle while using Ben-Wa Balls.

Butt-Plug

This toy is a dildo used for anal play. You can place it in the anus and leave it there while you have vaginal intercourse or oral or manual sex. The middle section is wider than the top and the bottom of the plug, and it's flared at the base to prevent the plug from getting lost in your rectum. (If it did, you'd require surgery to remove it.)

If you use a plug, start with a small one, be sure to use lots of lubrication, and insert the plug very slowly. Avoid altogether the plugs that are more than 4 inches long to prevent injury to your rectum.

Anal Beads

A series of round beads made of silicone or plastic are attached to each other by a string (nylon cord is the best). The beads, which come in different sizes, are inserted into the anus one by one and should be removed slowly and carefully. (Some people enjoy having the beads removed as they orgasm.) Before using anal beads made of plastic, be sure to file down any irregular areas with an emery board to keep from injuring yourself. As with all sex toys, be sure to use lots of lubricants and clean them regularly.

Aphrodisiacs

Throughout recorded history, people have searched for the perfect herb, drug, or food to increase sexual desire, arousal, and performance. In their quest, they've amassed an exhaustive list of substances that purportedly have aphrodisiac properties. Today, most have been proven to be ineffective; some have been shown to be dangerous; and others are so unusual that it's sometimes difficult to imagine that anyone was brave enough to be the first to try them. A list of the more unusual substances used throughout the ages includes bear's gallbladder, bird's nest soup, goat's testicle, crocodile kidneys, dried crocodile penis, and bull's urine.

Some ancient cultures thought that foods shaped like sexual organs were capable of adding zip to your sex drive. Phallic-shaped foods, such as carrots, asparagus, and cucumbers, and soft, moist foods or those shaped like the female genitals, such as oysters, clams, peaches, tomatoes, and eggs, were thought to light the sexual fires of men and women.

An infamous aphrodisiac, Spanish fly, may be harmful or deadly. Spanish fly comes from a dried beetle (*cantharis*). When you take it internally or apply it to the genitals, it causes prolonged erections and engorgement of the clitoris. Unfortunately, there have been deaths associated with the use of Spanish fly.

Herbs

For centuries, herbs have been used to improve all aspects of our sexuality, including desire, arousal, and performance or enjoyment of sex.

Black cohosh is a North American plant that has estrogenlike properties and increases blood flow to your pelvis, increasing your arousal and response to sexual stimulation.

Chasteberry is the dried fruit of the chaste tree. Despite its name, it's a libido booster: It increases *dopamine,* the neurotransmitter that increases your sexual desire and enjoyment, and decreases *prolactin,* the neurotransmitter that interferes with sexual desire.

Damiana is derived from a small shrub and has been used as a sexuality tonic for women. It has a soothing and calming effect that makes it easier for you to relax and enjoy sex. It may increase blood flow to your genitals, making it easier for you to achieve orgasm.

Fenugreek, a Mediterranean herb, dates back to ancient Egypt as an aphrodisiac. It increases libido and arousal, and it improves vaginal moisture in menopausal women.

Fo-ti, a Chinese herbal medicine, is thought to increase strength and blood flow to the genitals. It makes you more alert and energetic, and it increases your libido.

Garlic has been used for thousands of years to stir sexual appetite. It improves blood circulation and decreases blood pressure so that you have good blood flow to your genitals. When you take garlic, you also boost your energy and stamina—de rigueur for fantastic sex. Garlic is a natural treatment for chronic vaginal yeast infections.

Ginseng has been used for thousands of years as an aphrodisiac. It increases sexual desire and enhances performance by boosting energy and endurance.

Gotu kola increases your sex drive and sexual arousal and performance by increasing the blood flow to your genitals. Gotu kola is high in B vitamins, which are necessary to help fuel the increased energy required for satisfactory sex.

Muira puama, a Brazilian herb, increases your desire for sex and your arousal by increasing blood flow to your genitals. It may increase levels of testosterone, which is as important for women's sexuality as it is for men's.

Sarsaparilla, a vine found in the Caribbean, may increase your energy, sexual performance, and enjoyment of sex. It may increase libido in both women and men.

Yohimbine is an aphrodisiac made from the bark of the native African yohimbine tree. It is said to increase your libido and enhance your sexual performance because it increases levels of *norepinephrine,* a neurotransmitter that increases libido and sexual enjoyment. It also improves your mood and increases blood flow to your genitals. Yohimbine has been approved by the FDA (Food and Drug Administration) as a treatment for impotence and is available by prescription. Because of the risks of serious side effects, the herb should be used only under the supervision of a physician or other knowledgeable health-care provider.

Women frequently view herbs as a natural way to enhance sexuality. Herbs are strong medicine. They may be toxic alone, in certain dosages, or when combined with other herbs or medications. Before taking herbs, get professional help from an herbalist or a medical professional. When purchasing herbs, try to stick with companies known to provide quality products.

Food as Aphrodisiacs

Everything you eat or drink affects your motivation or desire for sex, your ability to respond to sexual stimulation, and the intensity of your response. Eating a variety of healthy foods is essential for a delicious sex life.

What you eat prior to sex can set the tone for the entire evening and make the difference between good sex and great sex. The meal should be light and stimulating to your taste buds. Keep in mind that high-fat foods decrease testosterone levels and decrease libido; foods high in sugar and carbohydrates and large amounts of tryptophan-containing foods like milk, cheese, and cream can make you drowsy; and too much alcohol will interfere with sexual performance and enjoyment.

For a romantic meal, choose foods that are noted for their reputed aphrodisiac effects. Prepare them in harmonious combinations, using cooking methods and seasonings that bring out the best flavors of the food. A sample menu might look like the one below:

Lover's Menu

Salad of wild greens, walnuts, apples, oil, and vinegar
Grilled salmon
Sautéed zucchini with mushrooms
Steamed carrots in lemon cream sauce
Brown rice pilaf with almonds
Strawberries dipped in chocolate
Parsley and mint sorbet (breath freshener)

Feasting in the Bedroom

Yes, food can be very stimulating in the bedroom. Feeding each other is an ancient technique used to increase arousal. Try a bowl of strawberries, grapes, or apple slices dipped in honey.

Make sure that whatever is placed in the vagina can also be easily and completely removed. In my practice, I have removed many edible items (grapes,

The Very Best Aphrodisiacs

❧ A mutually enjoyable and loving relationship

❧ An interesting and interested partner

❧ A healthy diet containing vitamins, minerals, water, and nutrients necessary for optimal health

❧ Regular exercise and a healthy body

❧ Sexual self-esteem (Feeling good about yourself helps you feel motivated to share the intimacy of sex with another person, or with yourself.)

❧ A healthy mind (Allows you to fantasize and be creative, increasing your desire for sex. Women-oriented erotic literature and videos can also be quite stimulating.)

berries, candy, and popcorn, to name a few) from vaginas. Avoid putting honey, whipped cream, and chocolate sauce inside the vagina, since they are difficult to remove and will increase your risk of a vaginal infection.

Romance Busters

Alcohol has gained the reputation of an aphrodisiac, and in small doses it may decrease your inhibitions and increase your relaxation enough to make you more desirous of sex. However, as little as one or two glasses of wine may make it harder for you to become aroused, and orgasm may be difficult or impossible to reach.

Recreational drugs are also thought to have aphrodisiac properties. Most illicit drugs are disastrous when it comes to great sex. In small doses marijuana may increase your libido, but in higher doses it can also cause mental distraction and make orgasm more difficult to achieve. Cocaine, heroin, and amphetamines may interfere with your desire and make it difficult to achieve orgasm.

Smoking has a sexy reputation but can decrease your arousal, energy, and stamina.

Part III

Taking Care
of
Yourself

Chapter 13

Sexercise: Working Out to Increase Your Sexuality

I'm sure you're aware of the many benefits of exercise. Regular exercise is good for your heart, helps you lose weight, and protects your bones. You've heard all the reasons you should work out, but are you aware that regular exercise can turn so-so lovemaking into fabulous can't-wait-to-tell-my-best-friend sex?

To understand why exercise is important, just look at what happens to your body during sex. As you become sexually excited, your heart begins to beat faster. Your heart rate increases further as sex continues and peaks during orgasm. Your blood vessels rush blood to your breasts, nipples, vagina, pelvis, skin, and muscles. Your blood pressure rises. You breathe faster, and as you near orgasm there is even a tendency to hyperventilate. The muscles of your abdomen, back, butt, and thighs get a good workout as you thrust and move during sex. And the muscles of your face, neck, legs, arms, and abdomen can spasm without your conscious control as you near and experience orgasm.

When we think of sex, we generally concentrate on what is going on in our erogenous zones, but as you can see, it's a total body experience—every system in your body is stimulated. If it is truly great sex, you can get quite a workout. Like any athletic pursuit, the better shape you're in, the better the experience is going to be. Getting in good physical shape will help you have more enjoyable sex.

What Exactly Will Exercise Do for Your Sex Life?

Exercise helps to improve your stamina or endurance, flexibility, and strength—all of which are important ingredients of great sex. People who exercise regularly desire sex more, have sex more frequently, tend to be more aroused, and enjoy sex more than those who don't exercise. It may even help you have more frequent and stronger orgasms.

Endurance

Endurance will enable you to have sex for as long as you wish. Remember, women need on average 12 minutes to reach orgasm; some of us need more than an hour of stimulation. If your candle is burning out after a few minutes, you may not be having the mind-blowing sex that you're entitled to. You can increase your stamina by including aerobic exercises in your daily routine. A mere 20 minutes of aerobic exercises a day can give you the endurance to hang with the best lovers in the world. Aerobic exercises include brisk walking, running, swimming, tennis, jumping rope, biking, and aerobic exercise classes. Try one of the many aerobic exercise tapes that are on the market—Tae-Bo or step aerobics, for example. They provide a great cardiovascular workout and improve your lower body strength.

Flexibility

Flexibility training enables you to assume any position you wish. It will give you the freedom to be creative in your sexual repertoire and get into the positions that give you the most stimulation of your most sensitive spots. You can wrap your legs around his back, put your heels on his shoulder, or assume any of the hundreds of positions described in the Kama Sutra. Even if you are not into gymnastic sex, enhanced flexibility will decrease the chances that you'll get muscle cramps, strains, or joint pain during sex. That kind of agility comes with regular stretching. You'll get the best results with 10–15 minutes of total body stretching at least four times a week. Yoga, Pilates, and T'ai Chi are excellent exercises to help improve your flexibility.

Strength

Strength training tones your muscles and helps them to function more efficiently, enabling you to assume any position that you desire. It also enables you to move your partner's body to the spot that gives you the most pleasure—and to hold it there as long as you need to. We sometimes shy away from strength training because we fear buffing up and looking like a male bodybuilder. The truth is that we women don't have the hormonal makeup to change our bodies that drastically—even with heavy weight lifting—so don't be afraid.

For the good of your sex life, add strength training to your schedule three to four times a week. Lifting weights, exercising with rubber bands, or doing pull-ups, chin-ups, and push-ups will help your body become firm and toned, and you'll feel stronger and more in charge of your body and your life. Don't forget the lower body—and the muscles you can't see. Strengthening your pelvic floor muscles can make it easier to achieve orgasms—and make them more intense.

Self-esteem

Exercise can improve your self-esteem by making you confident and comfortable with the way you look and feel. Often women worry about every bulge and soft spot on their bodies, hiding under the covers with the lights off for fear that their partner will discover their imperfections. And feeling bad about the way we look can sometimes interfere with our full enjoyment of the sexual experience.

Exercise can help you to lose those unwanted pounds and inches; you'll be firmer, more toned, and more adventurous. Exercising regularly will give you the courage to throw off the covers, keep the lights on, and maybe even do a striptease for your lover. Now *that* would get his attention.

Remember that sex itself is a form of aerobic exercise that can help you lose unwanted pounds. You'll burn up to 6 calories per minute. Just imagine what a daily dose of good sex can do for your body in a year.

Happiness

When you exercise, your body produces *endorphins,* often called "feel-good" hormones because they lift your mood and can temporarily relieve pain. Exercise can also help decrease stress, anxiety, and the blues. And if you feel good, you are more likely to desire and enjoy sex.

General Health Benefits

- Exercise strengthens your heart so you have the energy and stamina for a good night of sex. It also decreases your risks of heart disease.

- It makes your respiratory system stronger and more efficient so you'll be able to perform for longer periods of time without becoming breathless.

- Exercise (especially strength training) decreases LDL, or "bad cholesterol," which can clog your blood vessels. Keeping them open increases the blood flow throughout your body—including your vagina and pelvis—and improves your arousal, vaginal lubrication, and sexual enjoyment.

- Exercise decreases your risk of chronic illnesses such as high blood pressure and diabetes—diseases that can interfere with sexual performance and enjoyment.

- Exercise improves your sleep, and as you'll learn later, sleep improves your sex life.

- Exercise can relieve some of the symptoms of PMS (premenstrual syndrome), a true libido killer.

Exercise Tips

Before embarking on any exercise program, be sure to see your doctor for approval. Start slowly and gradually increase your workout as your strength and endurance improve. Allow several months of regular work before expecting a result.

Of course, it also helps if you can get your partner to exercise with you. It has been shown that men who exercise regularly have increased testosterone levels, better erections, more desire for sex, and happier partners. That information was enough for me to relieve my Nordic track of its clothes-hanging duties and encourage my husband to hop on board. Urge your partner to get into a fitness routine. It's good for his health—and the sight of his muscles while he's gliding on an exercise machine combined with the intoxicating effect of male sweat and pheromones may be enough to put a spark in your love life.

Don't overdo it, though. Too much exercising can have a negative effect on sex, leaving you too tired and sore for even a quickie. Very intense exercising, such as what some competitive athletes do, can cause a decrease in your estrogen levels, irregular or missed periods, vaginal dryness, and weak bones. Moderate exercise is best. *Consult your doctor if you notice any changes in your period after beginning a strenuous exercise program.*

Working Your Love Muscle

A strong "love muscle," the *pubococcygeus (PC),* can greatly improve your enjoyment of sex. This muscle stretches from your pubic bone to your *coccyx* (tailbone) and encloses your vagina and rectum like a sling. The nerve endings in the PC muscle are responsible for a lot of the sensations you feel during sexual intercourse. As the penis thrusts in and out of your vagina, the muscle stretches and relaxes, stimulating nerve endings and producing pleasurable sensations. It's this muscle that contracts rhythmically when most women reach orgasm.

The stronger and firmer the PC muscle, the more pleasure you can expect during intercourse, the greater your chance of orgasm, and the greater the intensity of the orgasm. Exercising your PC muscle increases blood flow to your pelvis, improving vaginal lubrication. A strong PC muscle makes your vagina feel tighter and enables you to grip and massage your partner's penis during intercourse, increasing his pleasure as well.

Kegel Exercises

The most common method used to strengthen the PC muscle are *Kegel exercises,* named for the gynecologist who devised them as treatment for women with urine incontinence. Patients who tried the exercises soon discovered that their enjoyment of sex and orgasms increased after several months of regular practice. Kegels make you more aware of sensations in your pelvis and increase your arousal.

Learning to do Kegels the correct way is not always easy because it is sometimes difficult to figure out exactly which muscles to contract. The easiest way for me to help my patients know what I'm talking about is by telling them that they can stop the flow of urine by contracting their PC muscle. To practice, sit on the toilet with your legs spread as far apart as possible to make sure you use only the PC muscle. When you begin to urinate, contract your pelvic floor muscles to stop the flow of urine. Practice contracting the muscle and stopping the flow of urine until you have a good sense of where the muscles are and how to tighten them.

Once you've identified the PC muscle, you can contract and release it anytime and anywhere, and do as many Kegels a day as you desire. Dr. Kegel used to recommend 300 contractions a day, but even if you don't do quite that many, establishing a daily routine will make it easier for you to remember to give your pelvic floor muscles the attention they need.

I recommend two sessions a day. Each session takes only a few minutes so they can easily fit into even the busiest schedule. Empty your bladder before you begin. Start by squeezing your PC muscle until you feel it tighten; hold the contraction for as long as you can. (In the beginning you may be able to hold the contraction for only a second or two.) Now relax the muscle for an equal number of seconds. Try to work up to holding the contraction for 10 seconds, then relaxing for 10 seconds. Repeat the tightening and relaxing for a set of 10–25 reps each session.

Be sure that you are not pushing down as you squeeze and aren't contracting the muscles of your abdomen, inner thigh, or butt. To ensure that you're contracting the right muscle, insert two clean fingers into your vagina and spread them apart in a V shape like a peace sign. When you squeeze your PC muscle, you should feel the walls of your vagina pressing against your fingers. In the beginning, the pressure may be very slight, but as your muscle becomes stronger, you'll be able to squeeze your two fingers together with the walls of your vagina.

To improve the endurance as well as the strength of your pelvic floor muscles, you'll want to add a series of rapid PC muscle contractions to your routine. This time squeeze and release your PC muscle once every second for a count of 5. Work up to a count of 20 contractions in 20 seconds. As your muscle becomes stronger you will be able to increase the speed of your contractions until your muscle moves in a kind of flutter. When you can do this, try it for a count of 5, rest for 15 seconds, and then repeat.

For advanced Kegels, try tightening your PC muscle, holding the contraction for 5 seconds, then pulling the muscle up a little tighter. You should be able to feel the increased tension in the muscle. Hold it there for another 5 seconds. Now tighten just a bit more and hold it there for another 5 seconds. Relax for 30 seconds. Repeat 5 times.

You can practice Kegels while lying, squatting, sitting, and standing—anywhere you want. But don't expect instant results. It can take several months of daily exercises before you notice a significant improvement in the strength of your PC muscle. Like any muscle, your PC muscle can get tired and sore after a vigorous workout—especially when you first start. If you have pain with sex or bowel movement, or just feel especially sore after a Kegel routine, take a few days off and start again with a less vigorous workout, gradually increasing the number of sets you do each day.

Weight Training for Your PC Muscle

Believe it or not, there's "weight-lifting" equipment for your vagina! At your pharmacy or doctor's office, in sex shops, and on the Net, you can find various kinds of devices that can assist you in exercising your PC muscle. Check the resource pages at the end of the book for details on where to find the following exercisers.

Kegelcisor

The Kegelcisor is a barbell for your PC muscle. I recommend that you begin your session by placing your Kegelcisor in warm water. (The Kegelcisor is metal, so it can be shockingly cold if it is not warmed up before being placed in your vagina.) Lie on your back with your head and shoulders supported on pillows and your knees bent. Lubricate your Kegelcisor and place it in your vagina. As you insert it, your PC muscle will automatically contract. Once you have it halfway in, contract your PC muscle to move the bar. The movements will be small initially. Hold, relax, and repeat for 20 counts twice a day. Another way to strengthen your muscles with the Kegelcisor is to place it in your vagina as before, but this time

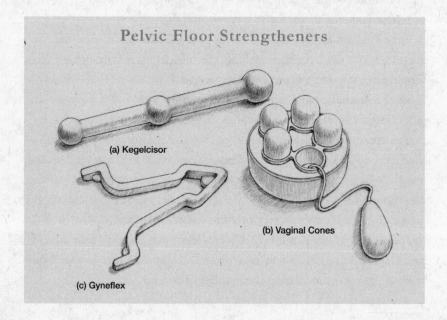

Pelvic Floor Strengtheners

(a) Kegelcisor

(b) Vaginal Cones

(c) Gyneflex

when you contract your PC muscle, you want to hold the squeeze while slowly pulling the Kegelcisor out of your vagina. Repeat this exercise at least 20 counts twice a day.

Vaginal Cones

Vaginal cones are another weight-lifting apparatus for your PC muscle. Cones can be purchased in your doctor's office, by prescription at a pharmacy or surgical supply store, or through the Internet. They come in sets of four or five cones all the same size but of increasing weights and shaped like tampons with a string for easy removal from your vagina. To begin, stand up, insert the lightest cone into your vagina, and hold it there by contracting your PC muscle. Now walk around the room with the cone in place. If you feel it slipping, replace it. Practice until you can hold the cone in place while walking for 15 minutes. During your next session, you can progress to the next heaviest cone. You can use the cones while showering or while busy about the house. To increase the intensity of your workout, walk briskly on the treadmill with the cone in place. Combining a workout with your vaginal cones in addition to your daily Kegel routine will give you strong PC muscles.

Gyneflex

The Gyneflex is a simple, plastic, wishbone-shaped resistance apparatus that helps strengthen your PC muscle like squeezing a hand spring strengthens the muscles of your hand. By providing resistance while you perform Kegels, the Gyneflex strengthens your PC muscle. To begin, lie on your back with your head and shoulders supported and your knees bent. Lubricate your Gyneflex with a water-based lubricant and insert it in your vagina. Once it is comfortably in place, contract your PC muscle and hold the squeeze as long as you can before relaxing. You will notice that the two arms of the Gyneflex come together when you contract your muscles. Work up to at least 20 repetitions per day. Gyneflex can be obtained through the Internet at www.gyneflex.com.

   NOTE: *Do not use vaginal cones, the Gyneflex, or the Kegelcisor while having your period, during pregnancy, or when you have an infection of your vagina or bladder.*

Other PC-Strengthening Techniques

Electrical Stimulation

Yeah, I know. The thought of electric current shooting through your pelvis sounds like the very last thing you'd want. However, doctors have used electrical stimulation of the pelvic floor muscles for many years. It is not painful and there are no known side effects. It's just a small electric current that, when applied to your pelvic muscles, causes them to contract. Electrical stimulation is especially useful if you aren't able to identify and contract your PC muscles or if your muscles are severely weakened. You can receive treatment in some doctor's offices or your doctor may be able to prescribe a safe portable unit for home use.

Neocontrol Therapy

Neocontrol therapy can be called an "automatic Kegel exercise machine." You sit in a special chair while highly focused magnetic fields aimed at the muscles of your pelvic floor cause the muscles to contract. Treatments last 20 minutes and are given twice a week for several weeks. It's not painful, has no known side effects, and is more efficient than Kegels. You don't have to do anything but sit there. Be warned: Some women have experienced orgasms while sitting in the chair—though this is not the manufacturer's intention! This treatment was approved by the FDA in 1998 but can be found in only a few doctors' offices.

Biofeedback

Biofeedback machines let you know when you are contracting your PC muscles, whether you are contracting the right muscle, and how strong those contractions are. A tamponlike probe is placed in your vagina, and as you do Kegel exercises, the probe records the strength of your contractions. Like the monitors on the exercise equipment in the gym, it enables you to follow your progress as your muscle becomes stronger. Seeing exactly how much effort you're making can motivate you to work harder.

Though biofeedback machines are most often used in doctors' offices, your physician can prescribe a small portable unit that you can use at home.

Full-Body Sexercises

Of course sexercise doesn't stop at the genitals; to be able to participate fully in exhilarating sex play, you will want your whole body to be in the best possible shape. You don't want to miss exercising any part of your body during your workout any more than you'd want your lover to miss stimulating any part of your body during lovemaking. Add these sex-specific exercises to your daily routine. *NOTE: If you have problems with your muscles or joints, or any other medical problems, please discuss any and all exercises with your doctor first.*

Sexercising Your Abdominals
Your abdominal muscles help to move your pelvis. To be a pro at the sexual moves described in Chapter 11, you've got to have strong, flexible abs.

Crunches
   Lie with your back flat on the floor and your knees bent. Place your hands behind your head, elbows out to the side. Slowly lift your head and

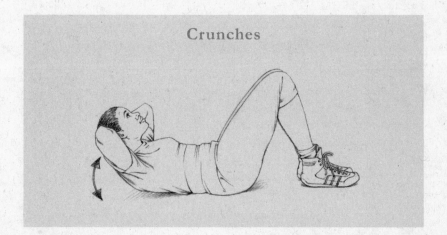

Crunches

shoulders using your abdominal muscles. Use your hands to support the back of your head—but don't jerk your neck—as you lift. Work up to at least 50 crunches per exercise session.

The Bicycle

Lie with your back flat on the floor and your knees bent. Place your hands behind your head, your elbows to the side. Raise your upper body until your shoulders are off the floor. "Pedal" as if riding a bicycle, raising your right knee to meet your left elbow halfway. Now alternate and touch your right elbow to your left knee. Repeat the cycle at least 25 times per exercise session.

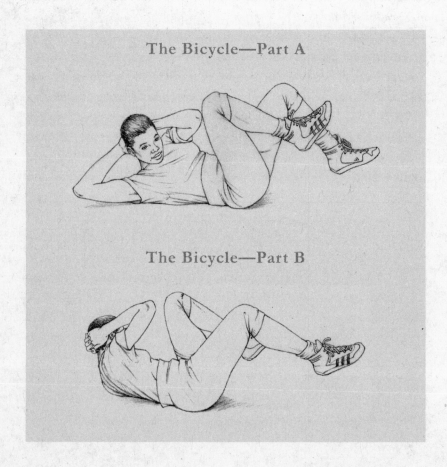

The Bicycle—Part A

The Bicycle—Part B

Leg Raises

Lie on your back on the floor. Place your hands under your buttocks to help flatten your lower back against the floor. Keeping your feet together and abs tight, raise your legs straight into the air. Now slowly lower your legs until they are about 6 inches from the floor. Hold for 5 seconds. Raise your legs again and repeat. Work up to 20 leg raises per session. *NOTE: Do not do this exercise if you have back problems.*

Sexercising Your Back

Your back is also important for moving your pelvis. To swivel your hips you need strong lower back muscles, and all the most pleasurable positions require your back to be flexible as well as strong.

The Cobra

Lie flat on your stomach with your forehead touching the floor. Place your hands flat on the floor and under your shoulders, with your elbows pointed back. Use your back muscles and arms to slowly raise your upper body as high as you can *comfortably,* keeping your abs, hips, and legs pressed to the floor. Hold this position for 5–10 seconds, then slowly lower your body to the floor. Repeat this exercise at least 20 times.

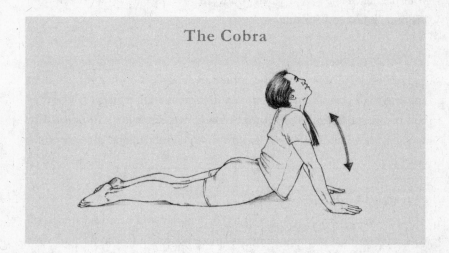

The Cobra

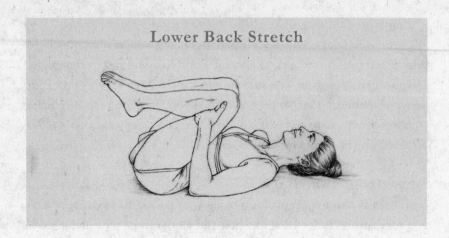

Lower Back Stretch

Lower Back Stretch

Lie on your back with your knees bent. Slowly bring your knees in to your chest. Grasp your thighs with your hands and hold the stretch for 20 seconds. Repeat.

Sexercising Your Inner Thighs

Contracting strong inner thigh muscles during intercourse can add to your arousal, increase friction to your clitoris, and create unique sensations for your partner. He'll love it when you wrap your legs around him and hold his body between your thighs.

The Stretch

Lie with your back flat on the floor. Raise your legs up straight, at a right angle to your body. Slowly open your legs, separating them as far apart as you comfortably can. Hold for 5 seconds. Repeat at least 10 times. You can use your hands to press down on your inner thighs for a stronger stretch.

Inner Thigh Lift

Lie on your left side. Place your left arm under your head and straighten your left leg. Bend your right knee and place your right foot in front of your left knee. Slowly raise your left leg until it is about 5 inches from the floor.

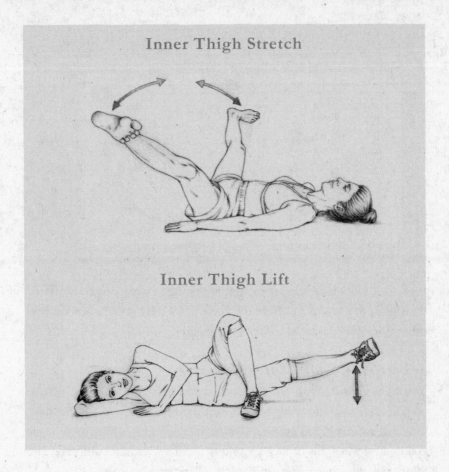

Inner Thigh Stretch

Inner Thigh Lift

Hold for a second, then lower. Repeat 10–20 times before turning to your right side.

Sexercising Your Outer Thighs

The hip joint is the most common area in which women develop discomfort during intercourse. The muscles surrounding your hip help support the joint, so developing strong outer thigh muscles can help prevent injury and develop the flexibility you need to move your hip joints.

Lateral Leg Lift

Lie on your side with your arm under your head. Bend your bottom leg and extend your top leg out straight from your body, starting with your

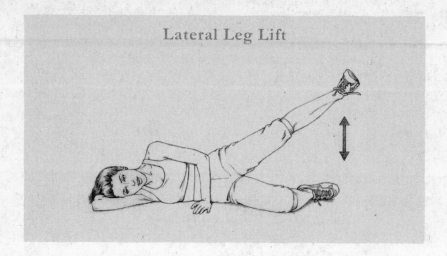

Lateral Leg Lift

foot on the floor. Slowly lift the top leg as high as you can comfortably, then lower to a few inches from the floor. Raise and lower. Repeat on your other side. Work up to 10–20 reps per session.

Sexercising Your Gluteal Muscles

You know a strong, well-toned butt is sexy. But did you know it can increase your arousal and enjoyment of sex? You need strong glutes for thrusting, grinding, swiveling, and gyrating your pelvis. Agile gluteal muscles can help you control where his penis goes, and squeezing your butt tightly and rapidly during intercourse or masturbation will increase your arousal.

Pelvic Tilt

Lie on your back on the floor, knees bent, feet flat on the floor and shoulder-width apart. Place your hands behind your head or at your sides. Lift your pelvis off the floor by tightening your gluteal muscles. Hold for a second, then lower your pelvis. Repeat the lifts at least 30 times each session. To increase the intensity, hold the lift for 10 seconds each time before relaxing.

Squat

Stand with your feet shoulder width apart. Keeping your back straight and your abdomen tucked in, lower your buttocks backward and into a sit-

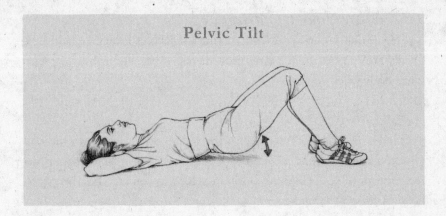

Pelvic Tilt

ting position. Hold for a second. Then squeeze your glutes as you raise your body back to the upright position.

To intensify your squats and give your inner thighs an additional work-out, place a large ball (soccer ball size) between your thighs. Squeeze your inner thigh muscles to keep the ball from falling. While squeezing the ball, perform the squat as previously described.

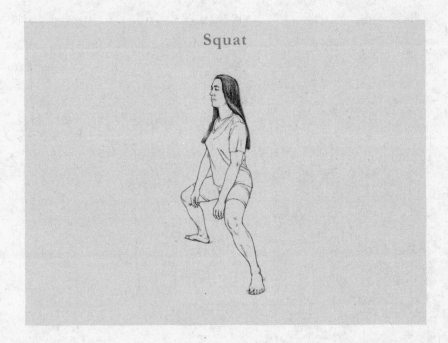

Squat

Sexercising Your Quadriceps

The big muscle group in the front of your thighs is called your quadriceps. Quads are important in pelvic movements, especially in moving your lower body when you are on top.

Wall Squat

Stand with your back flat against the wall. Slowly slide down the wall until you are in a sitting position with your feet firmly planted about two feet in front of you. Hold this position as long as you can and work up to holding it for 30 seconds.

Lunge Lap

Stand straight with your hands at your sides. Lunge forward with your right leg. Bring your left leg up to meet your right, and return to the standing position, squeezing your butt as you rise. Now lunge with your left leg. Alternate lunges until you have walked around the entire room.

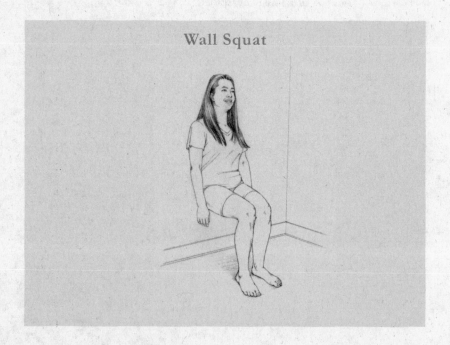

Wall Squat

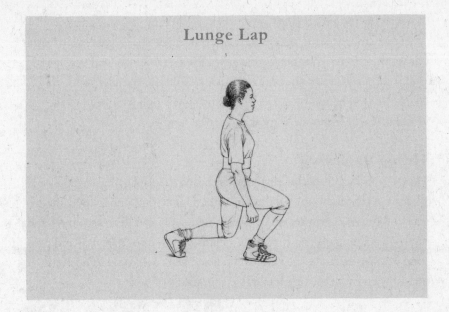

Lunge Lap

Sexercising Your Neck Muscles

We underestimate the importance of strong neck muscles. But if you've ever performed fellatio, you know that no matter what position you're in, your neck gets a workout. Giving him good oral sex can often leave you with a sore neck. Developing strong, flexible neck muscles will make it easier and more comfortable for you to find his hot spots. When exercising the neck, take it slow and easy, and build up your endurance over time. Be careful; it's quite easy to strain your neck. Stop immediately if you hear a popping sound or have pain while doing these exercises.

Front-to-Back Neck Stretches

Stand straight with your arms at your side, stomach tucked, shoulders back. Slowly drop your head forward as far as you can comfortably. Place both hands behind your head and *gently* pull your head forward and down toward your chest. Don't force or yank your neck. Hold for 3 seconds. Raise your head. Now slowly drop your head back and look up at the ceiling. Hold for 3 seconds. Raise your head. Repeat at least 10 times.

Side Neck Stretches

Stand straight with your hands at your sides. Place your right hand across the top of your head and on your left ear. Slowly and very gently pull your head toward your right shoulder. Hold the stretch for 3 seconds. Place your left hand on your right ear and slowly pull your head to the left side. Hold for 3 seconds. Repeat at least 10 times.

Heavy Breathing

Deep breathing, in specific rhythms, has been practiced by Eastern philosophers for centuries—in part because they have long understood the effects of breathing on sexuality. Breathing deeply can decrease stress and anxiety and prepare you for sex as well as increase your arousal and prolong your orgasm. Feeling calm and relaxed will enable you to be aware of and fully enjoy all of the pleasurable sensations of sex.

Belly Breathing

Lie flat on your back. Place one hand on your abdomen and close your eyes. Now breathe in slowly and deeply through your nose. As you breathe in, you should feel your abdomen rise as it fills with air. Hold the breath for a second, then exhale slowly and completely through your nose. You will notice your abdomen fall. Repeat at least 10 times. Gradually increase the number of breaths until you can comfortably practice belly breathing for 5–10 minutes. Practice belly breathing at least twice a day. You can also do it while comfortably seated. It's a great way to begin and end each day, a wonderful prelude to sex, and an aid in increasing your arousal during sex.

Chapter 14

In Control: Birth Control

One of my patients has unusual names for her children: One is her "diaphragm baby," another is her "rubber baby," and a third is her "Aspen baby." Babies one and two were conceived while using the obvious methods of contraception. Baby three was conceived when she went on vacation to Aspen and forgot her birth control pills.

We are lucky to have numerous methods of birth control, but none of them is perfect. Each has a possibility of failure: sometimes because we fail to use them as we should and sometimes because no method except abstinence is completely effective.

Conceiving a child when you are ready for one can be a wonderful and joyous experience. Finding yourself pregnant when you don't want to be, however, can be devastating. Protecting yourself from an unplanned pregnancy takes planning, and waiting until you're peeling off your panties is not the ideal time to start thinking about it. Taking the time to explore the available choices and deciding which is the best for you are well worth the effort.

How to Find the Best Method of Contraception

You will need to consider the following:

- Is the method safe?

- How well does it protect me from pregnancy?

- Will this method protect me from sexually transmitted infections?

- Is it easy to use, and will I be able to use it correctly?

- Will I use this method every time I have sex?

- Do I want to get pregnant in the future? When?

- Can I afford to use this method?

- Will this method interrupt the flow of sex? Will that affect my motivation to use the method?

- How does my partner feel about the method?

As you consider the best method of birth control, give as much consideration to your need to prevent sexually transmitted infections as you do to birth control. STIs can cause anything from annoying discomfort to infertility to death, and few of the available contraceptives provide adequate protection. If you are not in a mutually monogamous relationship or you and your partner have not been tested to ensure that you are infection-free, you may need to use a condom along with your chosen method of birth control.

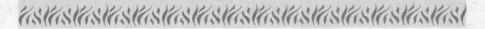

You're in Charge!

As a woman, you have the right to control your fertility: how many children you have and when you have them. I have found that some young women harbor the romantic notion that since it takes two to make a baby, two will completely share all of the consequences and responsibilities of any unintended pregnancy. But this is sometimes not the case. If you find yourself unexpectedly in the family way, it will be you who will have to cope with much if not all of the physical and emotional consequences of your decision to end or continue the pregnancy. It will be you who gains the weight, vomits, and gets the headaches, back pain, leg cramps, varicose veins, sore breasts, stretch marks, hemorrhoids, and discomforts of labor and delivery.

Carefully consider all of the available options for birth control and decide which method is right for you and your lifestyle. Discuss your options with your mate and doctor. In the end, the decision is yours to make. It's your body.

Birth Control and Sexuality

In many ways, birth control can be a huge boost to your sexuality. Lifting the fear of pregnancy may make you more desirous of sex, more relaxed and able to respond, and freer to try new sexual techniques. However, aside from abstinence, no method is 100 percent effective, and pregnancy concerns can sometimes dampen your full enjoyment of intercourse. Many of the side effects of various methods (such as sore breasts and possible weight gain) may have a definite effect on your sex drive. Overall, though, if you feel comfortable with your method of birth control, you will be much more relaxed and therefore sexier.

Methods from A to Z

Now that we know what doesn't work, let's take a comprehensive look at what does. Here, we'll explore different birth control methods and what you can do if your contraception fails. We'll examine each method carefully, taking a look at how it works, how effective it is, how you use it, the advantages and disadvantages, and for whom each method is best. You'll notice that I describe failure rates during the first year of use. This is because women are more likely to make a mistake when they're first learning to use a contraceptive or incorporate it into their lifestyle, so the chance that they'll get pregnant is higher. The risk typically goes down during subsequent years of use.

This chapter will give you information to help you have an informed conversation with your partner and gynecologist about what type of contraception is best for you.

Abstinence

For some of us, abstinence means saying no to any intimate acts. For others, abstinence means avoiding only vaginal intercourse. True abstinence requires saying no to vaginal intercourse, anal intercourse, and any activity that may place sperm near your vagina.

How does it work?

If you plan to use abstinence as your method of contraception, you will need to avoid not only vaginal intercourse but also "outercourse," anal sex, and any other activity that might place sperm anywhere near your vagina. Sperm released near your vagina are capable of swimming up your vagina and into your uterus.

How effective is it?

Complete abstinence is the only method that is 100 percent effective in preventing pregnancy.

Myths About Birth Control and Pregnancy

Many myths about pregnancy and birth control abound. Most of these myths float between teens, the group most at risk for an unintended pregnancy. Let's look at some of the most common.

〰 **You cannot get pregnant standing up.** Standing up while having sex will not protect you against pregnancy. Gravity will not make the sperm slide out of your vagina. Sperm swim up and into your uterus within minutes after your partner ejaculates.

〰 **You cannot get pregnant the first time you have sex.** It only takes once, and the first time counts! You must be prepared every time you have sex.

〰 **You cannot get pregnant during your period.** If you have short menstrual cycles, meaning your periods arrive every 21–24 days, it is possible for you to ovulate while you are still bleeding.

〰 **You cannot get pregnant before you have your first period.** Many adolescents believe this myth and place themselves at risk for pregnancy. The truth is that you can ovulate before your first period and become pregnant.

〰 **Douching after sex is a good method of birth control.** Immediately after your partner ejaculates, sperm swim rapidly up and into your cervix and uterus. In other words, by the time you douche, the horse is already out of the barn.

〰 **You can only get pregnant if he comes in your vagina.** You can become pregnant if he ejaculates anywhere near your vagina. Sperm are capable of swimming up your vagina and into your uterus.

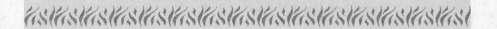

How do you use it?

Avoid all activities that might place sperm in or near your vagina. Masturbation, kissing, touching, and massage are reasonable outlets for sexual expression. If you have a partner, make sure that he understands (in advance of any intimacy) your decision to abstain from sex.

What are the advantages?

If you have no intimate contact with another person, you are protected against sexually transmitted infections (STIs) as well as pregnancy. Abstinence has no side effects, is reversible, and free.

What are the disadvantages?

Abstinence takes self-control and commitment.

Who shouldn't use this method?

Don't use this method if you find it difficult to say "no." A moment of weakness can lead to an unplanned pregnancy.

Who should use this method?

Abstinence is for you if you can easily say "no." If you are in a relationship, it helps if your partner agrees with your decision to abstain from sex. But in the end, you are in charge of what you do sexually.

Birth Control Pill (Oral Contraceptives)

Birth control pills are made of two hormones: estrogen and progestin. There are many different brands of birth control pills, but they all work the same way. The most commonly used pills are low dose and contain 30 or 35 mcg of estrogen. Newer birth control pills contain as little as 20 mcg of estrogen. And all birth control pills contain one of several different progestins.

In most pill packs, you will find equal amounts of estrogen and progestin in each of the 21 active (hormone-containing) pills. These are called *monophasic* pills. Some pill packs contain an additional 7 pills that do not contain hormones. Some packs will have pills that vary in their dosage of progestin or estrogen during the cycle. These pills are called *triphasic* and are usually different colors.

What Happens If I Miss a Pill?

If you miss a pill, take it as soon as you remember and take the next pill at the usual time. It is okay to take two at a time, but expect some nausea to follow. Continue to take the remaining pills at the right time.

If you have sex during the seven days following skipping one pill, use a backup method like a condom or diaphragm. After seven days of taking the pill correctly, you are once again protected against pregnancy. Don't be surprised, though, if you have spotting or bleeding after skipping one pill. And the spotting may continue until you start the next pack of pills.

If you miss more than one pill, take the last missed pill as soon as you remember, then take the next pill at the usual time. You do not need to take the other missed pills. Continue the rest of the pack as usual and use another method of contraception for the rest of this cycle of pills. You can expect to have some spotting or bleeding after you miss the pills, and this bleeding may continue until you start the next pack.

If you vomit within 2 hours after taking your pill, be sure to take another active pill.

How does it work?

The pill prevents pregnancy by stopping your *ovulation,* the production of an egg each month. It also thickens the mucus in your cervix so that it is difficult for sperm to enter your uterus.

How effective is it?

Birth control pills are very effective when taken properly. If you take your pills every day at the same time each day, your chances of becoming pregnant are very small, about 0.1 percent. However, most of us are not perfect users of the pill and have a slightly higher risk of pregnancy, about 5 percent in the first year of use.

Call Your Doctor If You Are on the Pill and:

≋ You have severe abdominal pain.

≋ You have severe chest pain or shortness of breath.

≋ You have a severe headache.

≋ You have a change in your eyesight (blurred vision or loss of vision).

≋ You have severe pain in your leg, especially if you also have swelling and increased warmth in the leg.

How do you use it?

You can start your pills on the first Sunday after you start your period, whether you are still bleeding or not. Another option is to start your pills on the first day of your period. Use a backup method—like the condom—the first week after you start taking the pill. After a week of taking the pills correctly, you are protected against pregnancy. Choose a time of day that will make it easy for you to remember to take your pill. I often tell patients to take the pill with food to decrease the nausea that you sometimes have when starting, so choose the meal that you are less likely to skip and take it with that meal every day. It is very important to take your pill at the same time every day; taking them at different times will increase your risk of pregnancy and cause you to have spotting and irregular bleeding. Even a 2-hour difference from one day to the next may cause spotting.

Your periods may become very light while using the pill—sometimes only a pink or brown spot on your pad or tampon. Some months you may see no signs of blood at all. If you have taken your pills every day at the same

Breast Feeding and Birth Control

Lactacting women have less than a 1 percent chance of becoming pregnant the first six months after giving birth if they feed their babies exclusively with their breasts—no bottles allowed—and their menses has not returned.

When the baby sucks on your nipples, a hormone called *prolactin* is released from your brain and causes milk to come down; as an added bonus, it also stops your ovulation. Unfortunately this rule, like all rules, does not apply to every woman, and some will ovulate anyway. So use a method of contraception if you do not want to get pregnant right away.

time each day, you are unlikely to be pregnant. Continue to take your pills as usual, but take a pregnancy test or arrange to see your doctor.

What are the advantages?

Birth control pills are very effective and allow you to have spontaneous sex anytime and as often as you like without concerns about pregnancy.

Pills are easily reversible. If you want to get pregnant, you just stop taking them. Traditionally, doctors have told patients to wait three months before getting pregnant after stopping the pill. Studies have shown that there is no harm to you or the baby if you get pregnant right after stopping the pill. Don't be surprised if it takes a few months for you to start having regular menstrual periods.

What are the disadvantages?

Birth control pills do not protect you against sexually transmitted infections. If you are at risk, it is important to use a condom in addition to the pill.

Common minor side effects include mild headaches, breast tenderness, and weight gain. Though every woman worries about the possibility of weight gain, as many women lose as gain weight while taking the pill. If you gain weight, consider changing your pill, increase your exercise, and watch what you eat. Though rare, there is a very small risk of a serious complication such as heart attack, stroke, or blood clots while taking the pill. Smoking while taking the pill increases your chance of a serious complication. Make sure you know the warning signs and when to call your doctor. You may notice mood changes or depression while taking the pill. Changing to a very low-dose, monophasic pill may brighten your moods.

Medications taken for epilepsy and some antibiotics (ampicillin, doxycycline, and tetracycline) may make the pills less effective. Use a backup method of birth control while taking these medicines and for seven days after stopping the medications.

The primary disadvantage for most women is that you must remember to take the pill every day, even if you are not having sex very often.

How does this method affect your sexuality?

Birth control pills have been shown to decrease free testosterone levels (the male hormone) and may dampen your desire. If you find that your desire for and enjoyment of sex have taken a nosedive, speak to your doctor about changing the type of pill (low-dose, monophasic is better) or your method of contraception. Pills may also cause your vagina to be drier, increasing your discomfort during sex.

Cervical Cap

The cervical cap is a small latex cup that is placed over your cervix before sex. Cervical caps come in four sizes and must be fitted by a doctor or nurse.

How does it work?

It fits snugly over your cervix and does not allow sperm to enter your uterus.

How effective is it?

The cap is more effective in women who have not had children than in women who have had a vaginal birth. If you have not had children, your risks of pregnancy the first year of use is between 9 percent and 20 percent. If you have had children, your risks may increase to 26–40 percent the first year of use.

How do you use it?

Place a teaspoon of spermicidal cream inside the dome of the cervical cap. Slide the cap into your vagina and over your cervix. Slide your finger around the edges of the cap to make sure that your cervix is completely covered. You can leave the cap in place for up to 48 hours, and you must leave it in for at least 8 hours after your last act of intercourse. *NOTE: Leaving the cap in for 48 hours will increase the likelihood of developing vaginal discharge and odor.*

What are the advantages?

There is no need to interrupt sex to insert the cap, and you can have intercourse as many times as you want in the 48 hours that the cap is in place. It is small and usually not noticed by your partner.

What are the disadvantages?

To properly use the cap, you must feel comfortable placing your fingers in your vagina and know where your cervix is and what it feels like.

The cervical cap does not protect you from sexually transmitted infections, and, like the diaphragm, you may notice that you have more frequent urinary tract (bladder) infections. Because it sits tightly on your cervix, you may have an increased risk of abnormal pap smears and should have a pap smear done three months after beginning to use a cervical cap.

How does this method affect your sexuality?

The cap is small and comfortable for you and your partner during intercourse. The cap must be positioned beforehand, so some planning is necessary.

Male Condom

Male condoms are sheaths placed over the head and shaft of the penis. The condom has increased in popularity because it is the best way to protect yourself from HIV and other sexually transmitted infections.

How does it work?

Condoms block the penis from your vagina and cervix. When he ejaculates, the sperm are trapped inside the condom and cannot reach your vagina or the waiting egg.

How effective is it?

If you use condoms correctly and every time you have sex, you have a small risk of pregnancy the first year of use, about 3 percent. Most of us do not always use them correctly or each time we have sex, and the risk of pregnancy in the real world increases to about 14 percent.

How do you use it?

For a condom to be effective, you must use it every time you have sex, and it must be rolled onto his penis from the beginning of sexual intimacy.

What are the advantages?

Condoms are inexpensive and easy to find in pharmacies, restrooms, and gas stations. You can find a virtual cornucopia of condoms on the Internet (my favorite site is www.condomania.com) as well as in shops and mail-order catalogs that sell sex toys. Unless you are allergic to latex, there are few if any side effects with the use of condoms. NOTE: If you develop a rash, itching, or wheezing after using latex condoms, you may have a latex allergy. Avoid any further contact with latex condoms or gloves. You can safely use the polyurethane or natural lambskin condoms for birth control. The intensity of sensations for some men is decreased, enabling them to stay harder longer, and condoms may help a man with premature ejaculation to go the distance.

What are the disadvantages?

Just when things are getting hot and heavy, you have to stop to put on the condom. For some couples, this can be annoying and in some cases leads to a bad decision to skip the condom "just this one time."

Learn to include the condom in your foreplay. As you roll down the condom with one hand, the other can massage the base of his penis,

Condoms, Rubbers, and Prophylactics: Choosing the Right Condom

I encourage women in my practice to take the responsibility of buying the condoms. That way you won't find yourself naked before you discover that he forgot to pick some up. For some of us, trying to stop at this point is like a skier trying to brake during an avalanche.

There are hundreds of condoms to choose from. You can find them in different sizes, colors, textures, flavors, and materials.

Sizes

Condoms come in three sizes: snug-fitting, regular, and large. Don't bother asking him what size he wears. And sizes are not written on the outside of most condom packages. Keep a variety of condoms handy so you always have just the right size. Try different sizes and brands until you find the one that gives you both the most pleasure.

Materials

Condoms may be made from latex (rubber), the intestines of lambs (natural lambskin), and polyurethane and newer plastics. Latex, natural, and plastic condoms will protect you equally well against pregnancy. But unlike the other two, the natural lambskin condom does not protect you against viral infections like HIV.

Latex condoms are the least expensive and the easiest to find in your local pharmacy. All lubricants used with latex condoms must be water based. Any oil-based lubricant can damage the latex. NOTE: *Whipped*

continued

cream and massage oil will damage latex condoms. And when you are using a vaginal cream for a yeast infection, choose a polyurethane condom.

Natural lambskin condoms are more expensive and wider than regular-sized latex condoms. Some men may have increased sensitivity while using natural condoms, and many women find the feel of lambskin condoms to be more pleasurable. Use them only if you are certain that you don't need protection against sexually transmitted infections.

Polyurethane condoms are twice as expensive as latex condoms and have no odor or taste (good for oral sex). They can be used with oil-based or water-based lubricants, but you may find them more difficult to slip on, and they can be noisy during sex. Many men and women find them to be sensitive, quite pleasurable, and worth the extra cost.

Condom Textures and Flavors

Condoms can be found with studs or ribbing to give you and your partner more pleasure. They come in many flavors, such as mint and cherry, though mint is the only flavor that is FDA approved.

Condoms come rolled up in individual packages. They may be dry or they may contain a water-based lubricant or nonoxynol-9, a spermicide. Recent studies have suggested that condoms lubricated with nonoxynol-9 may increase your risks of contracting HIV. (Nonoxynol-9 causes irritation of your vagina and exposes you to infection with the HIV virus.) Though it is better to use a plain, lubricated condom, using one with spermicide is better than no condom at all.

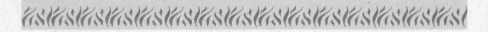

scrotum, or inner thigh. Some women have even mastered the art of rolling on a condom with their lips and tongue. Practice rolling a condom on a cucumber before intimacy.

Using a condom for contraception requires advance planning. You must have a condom with you at all times. Having dozens on your bedside table does you no good when you are slipping under the sheets in his apartment.

Condoms are not fully effective in protecting you from herpes or genital warts, as your partner may carry either infection at the base of his penis or scrotum, two areas not covered by the condom.

Condoms can break or slip off during intercourse, increasing your chances of pregnancy. You can decrease the chances of breakage by using lots of lubricant outside the condom and in your vagina. Condoms can cause your natural lubrication to dry out prematurely and can also cause vaginal dryness, pain, and swelling. *If the condom breaks during intercourse call your doctor and request emergency contraception.*

How does this method affect your sexuality?

Some men and women feel that intimacy is decreased when using a condom. Since the penis has to be withdrawn almost immediately after he ejaculates, the closeness and euphoria you feel after orgasm can be interrupted.

Many men complain of decreased sensation during sex with a condom. You can increase his pleasure by placing a few drops of water-based lubricant in the tip of the condom before rolling the condom onto the penis. The lubricant causes the condom to fit more snugly on the head of his penis and to move more naturally. Two new condom brands designed to give him maximum sensitivity, InSpiral and Pleasure Plus, are wonderful.

Female Condom: The Reality Female Condom

The Reality condom is a soft, lubricated, polyurethane pouch that is placed in your vagina before sex. It has two rings: one at the closed end of the pouch to make insertion easier and one at the open end of the pouch.

How does it work?

The female condom covers the walls of your vagina as well as part of your vulva. Like the male condom, it blocks his sperm from your vagina and cervix.

How effective is it?

There is a small risk of pregnancy if you use the female condom correctly and each time you have sex, about 5 percent in the first year of use.

Since most of us aren't perfect users of birth control, the typical user failure rate is closer to 21 percent.

How do you use it?

The female condom is placed in your vagina up to 8 hours before you have sex. Push the inner ring high into your vagina against your cervix. The outer ring should rest on your labia. While holding the outer ring of the condom against your labia with one hand, carefully guide his penis into the center of the ring and condom. Remove the condom after intercourse and throw it away. *Do not reuse female condoms.*

What are the advantages?

Like the male condom, the female condom is effective in protecting you against sexually transmitted infections, including HIV. Because the female condom also shields you from the base of his penis and scrotum, the female condom may provide better protection from infections like herpes and genital warts, and it gives you an option if your partner refuses to use the male condom.

It gives women an increased degree of control over contraception and self-protection from STIs. It comes in one size and can be purchased in your local pharmacy without a prescription.

What are the disadvantages?

The female condom costs three to four times more than the male condom. It is large, unattractive, and can be noisy during sex. The manufacturer suggests that you try the female condom at least three times before making a decision.

How does this method affect your sexuality?

Though it is pleasurable for most couples, some men and women may find the female condom uncomfortable. Placing additional lubricant inside and outside the condom may increase the pleasure for you and your partner.

Depo-provera

Depo-provera, also known as the "shot," is a progestin hormone that is given by injection.

How does it work?

Depo-provera prevents pregnancy by stopping your ovulation. It also thickens your cervical mucus so that sperm cannot get past your cervix.

How effective is it?

Depo-provera is highly effective, and your risk of becoming pregnant with proper use is 0.3 percent.

How do you use it?

Your doctor will write a prescription for Depo-provera and give you the injection in your arm or buttocks. You will need to return to the office every three months for a repeat injection.

What are the advantages?

Your chances of becoming pregnant while using Depo-provera are very small; there are few side effects; and you only need treatment four times a year. It is convenient and doesn't interfere with spontaneity.

What are the disadvantages?

Depo-provera does not protect you from sexually transmitted infections. The most common complaint of women using Depo-provera is irregular bleeding or spotting, which is most common during the first year of use. After the first year, you can expect to have no periods at all.

You may gain a few pounds when starting Depo-provera. Watching your calories, avoiding foods laden with salt, and exercising daily will help keep unwanted pounds in check.

It may take several months for your period to return after you decide to discontinue Depo-provera.

How does this method affect your sexuality?

Depo-provera lifts the fear of pregnancy and allows you to have more enjoyable sex. You can have sex when and as often as you want to.

If the shot makes you tired or moody, causes you to spot irregularly or gain weight, gives you headaches or sore breasts, you can expect your desire for sex to take a nosedive. If they occur at all, most of these side effects are temporary.

Diaphragm

The diaphragm is a soft, dome-shaped, latex cup that is placed in your vagina before sex.

How does it work?

The cap covers your cervix, holds spermicidal cream near your cervix, and prevents sperm from entering your uterus.

How effective is it?

If you use the diaphragm correctly each and every time you have sex, your chances of getting pregnant are 6 percent. The typical failure rate in the first year of use is 20 percent.

How do you use it?

You can place the diaphragm in your vagina up to 6 hours before sex. Before inserting the diaphragm, place about two teaspoons of contraceptive cream in the dome of the diaphragm. Slide the diaphragm far back into your vagina and use your finger to make sure that your cervix is completely covered by the diaphragm. The diaphragm should not be removed until at least 6 hours after your last act of intercourse to be certain that all sperm have been killed. If you plan to have sex after the 6-hour window has passed, use an applicator to place more contraceptive cream in your vagina. You will need to add more contraceptive cream before each act of intercourse. After you remove the diaphragm, wash it with soap and warm water, rinse well, and air-dry before placing it back in the case. Also, check for holes or cracks after each use. *If you find a hole after having sex, call your doctor for a prescription for emergency contraception.* Replace your diaphragm at least every two years.

Learning to use the diaphragm correctly takes practice. In the beginning you may become frustrated as the diaphragm goes sailing across the bathroom floor instead of into your vagina. Practice inserting and removing the diaphragm before leaving your doctor's office with a prescription, and several more times at home before using it during sex.

What are the advantages?

The diaphragm is safe, has few side effects, reduces your risks of infection with gonorrhea and chlamydia, and decreases your chances of having an abnormal pap smear.

A diaphragm gives you control of your birth control method.

What are the disadvantages?

The diaphragm must be fitted by your doctor or a nurse, and you need a prescription. You must use the diaphragm every time that you have sex, and sometimes that means you must carry your diaphragm with you at all times or have a diaphragm in more than one location.

It does not protect you against many STIs, including the HIV virus, and diaphragm users suffer from more urinary tract infections and vaginal infections than other women. Contraceptive creams may be the main culprits, but changing the size of your diaphragm sometimes helps decrease bladder infections.

Your partner may complain that he feels the diaphragm during sex. If so, ask your doctor to check the size of your diaphragm and change to a diaphragm with a softer rim, such as the flat or coil-spring types. You might also try changing the positions you use during sex.

How does this method affect your sexuality?

There is loss of spontaneity when using the diaphragm. Unless you know in advance exactly when you will be having intercourse, you will have to interrupt sex play to insert the diaphragm before intercourse.

Many think that the spermicide used with a diaphragm tastes awful. So if you enjoy oral sex you will need to interrupt the natural flow of sex to insert your diaphragm before intercourse. If your partner is willing, you can make insertion of the diaphragm a part of foreplay and ask your partner to insert it.

Intrauterine Device (IUD)

An IUD is a small thin device that is placed in your uterus to prevent pregnancy.

How does it work?

There are three types of IUDs. The Copper-T IUD (Paragard) is made of plastic and copper and works by preventing his sperm from fertilizing your egg. Paragard gives up to 10 years of protection. The second type, the Progestasert, is made of plastic and contains a progesterone-type hormone. Progestasert releases the hormone and changes the lining of your uterus, making it difficult for pregnancy to occur. This IUD must be changed yearly. A new IUD, the Mirena, releases a progesterone-type hormone and provides 5 years of protection.

How effective is it?

The risk of pregnancy with the Copper-T IUD is less than 1 percent. The risk of pregnancy with the Progestasert is slightly higher at 1.5 percent. And the risk with Mirena is 0.5 percent.

How do you use it?

Your doctor will insert the IUD into your uterus. The string attached to the base of the IUD will hang from your cervix and can be felt in your vagina. You will need to check for the IUD string after each menstrual period to make sure that the IUD has not been expelled from your uterus.

What are the advantages?

Though there are many misconceptions about the IUD, it is very safe if you are in a mutually monogamous relationship, and it can be easily inserted and removed by your doctor.

Considering that the Copper-T IUD remains effective for 10 years, it is an inexpensive method of contraception. The Progestasert and Mirena IUDs may make your periods lighter and less painful.

What are the disadvantages?

The IUD does not protect you from sexually transmitted infections, so it is not a good choice if you or your partner has multiple sex partners and you are not using condoms. You may increase your risks of pelvic infections that can lead to infertility.

Intrauterine devices may change your bleeding patterns. Your periods may be heavier and more painful, and you may have spotting between periods. *Be sure to see your doctor for any changes in your periods.* If you have never had a baby, the IUD may not be a good method for you.

Lunelle

Lunelle is an injection of estrogen and progestin (the hormones found in combination birth control pills) that prevents pregnancy.

How does it work?

Like the birth control pills that you take by mouth, Lunelle stops your ovulation every month.

How effective is it?

If you get your injections on time and every month, your chances of becoming pregnant are almost zero.

How do you use it?

You will need to go to your doctor's office every month for the injection. The first injection is given within the first 5 days after you start your period. You will need to repeat the injection every 28 days.

What are the advantages?

Lunelle is highly effective. There is no need to remember to take pills, and as long as you get the injection on time, you are nearly fully protected from pregnancy. Lunelle appears to have few side effects and is easily reversible.

What are the disadvantages?

Lunelle must be given by injection every month. A visit to a doctor's office or clinic is necessary to get the shot.

Lunelle does not protect you from sexually transmitted infections.

Emergency Contraception

No matter how careful you might be, occasionally accidents do happen. The condom might break, or you might find yourself basking in the afterglow of orgasm when you realize that you forgot your diaphragm. If you find yourself in need of emergency contraception, call your doctor as soon as possible.

There are two types of emergency contraception: hormones and intrauterine devices.

Hormones: The Morning-After Pill

To be effective, hormones—combined birth control pills or progesterone-only pills—must be taken within 72 hours of unprotected sex. The sooner after sex the hormones are consumed, the greater your chance of preventing pregnancy.

The most common oral contraceptive to prescribe for emergency contraception is Ovral. You will need to take 2 Ovral tablets (or another pill containing 50 mcg of estrogen) within 72 hours of unprotected sex and another 2 Ovral tablets 12 hours later. Low-dose pills are also effective, but more pills are needed to provide the needed dosage of hormones (4 pills containing 35 mcg of estrogen or 5 pills containing 20 mcg of estrogen). A new kit, Preven, contains 4 pills and a pregnancy test. You will need a prescription from your doctor to receive Preven.

If you can't take estrogen, mini pills (containing progesterone only) may be prescribed instead of combined pills. The most common mini pill used for this purpose is Ovrette. You will need to take 20 pills as soon as possible and another 20 pills 12 hours later. A new morning-after pill, Plan-B, also contains only progestin. Two pills containing a high dose of progestin are included in Plan-B, one to be taken immediately and the second 12 hours later.

Hormonal emergency contraception stops or delays your ovulation and

continued

may also change the lining of your uterus so that pregnancy does not take place. If the pills are taken properly, your risk of pregnancy is low, between 0.5 and 2.5 percent.

The most common side effects (of the combined pills, not the mini pills or Plan-B) are nausea and vomiting. Your doctor may prescribe another medication to prevent nausea. If not, take the pills with food and eat frequent small meals for the next 24 hours. Ginger tea and peppermint may help to settle your stomach.

Your period may come early, on time, or a little bit late. If your period is more than seven days late, take a pregnancy test.

Copper-Containing IUD

If you had unprotected intercourse more than 72 hours but less than five days before requesting emergency contraception, your doctor might suggest placing an intrauterine device (IUD) in your uterus. A copper-containing IUD will prevent fertilization or change the lining of your uterus so that pregnancy does not take place.

How does this method affect your sexuality?

There is almost zero chance of pregnancy so you may find that your libido and enjoyment of sex increase. Like the birth control pill, if you become moody, have breast tenderness, or experience increased vaginal dryness, your enjoyment of sex may decrease.

Mini Pill

Mini pills are progesterone-only pills taken to prevent pregnancy.

How does it work?

The mini pill may stop ovulation. It also blocks sperm from your cervix and changes the lining of your uterus to inhibit pregnancy.

How effective is it?

If the mini pill is taken correctly, the risk of pregnancy while using it is 0.5 percent.

How do you use it?

The mini pill must be taken every day, and unlike the traditional birth control pill, there is no seven-day break. It must be taken at the same time each day to keep your hormone levels steady. Taking it at odd hours will increase not only spotting but also the likelihood of pregnancy.

What are the advantages?

The mini pills can be taken by women who can't take estrogen and those who are breast feeding. They are highly effective and have few side effects.

What are the disadvantages?

Mini pills may change your bleeding patterns. You may have irregular spotting during the first few months of taking the mini pills or you may lose your period entirely. Mini pills may cause breast tenderness, mild depression, or weight gain, and they do not protect against STIs.

How does this method affect your sexuality?

The side effects that sometimes accompany mini pills can put a damper on your desire and enjoyment of sex.

Norplant

Norplant is a system of six small plastic capsules containing a progestin similar to the natural progesterone that you produce in your body.

How does it work?

Small amounts of progestin are released from the capsules daily for five years. Norplant stops your ovulation and makes your mucus so thick that sperm cannot get to your uterus. It may also make the lining of your uterus thin, so pregnancy cannot take place.

How effective is it?

Norplant is a very effective method of birth control and has a failure rate of only .05 percent.

How do you use it?

Your doctor will make a tiny incision and insert the six capsules under your skin. The capsules should be inserted in the first few days after you start your period and become effective after three days. The capsules are removed in five years, or sooner if you decide to get pregnant.

What are the advantages?

Norplant is one of the most effective methods of birth control, providing years of protection with few side effects and is easily reversible.

You may have less bleeding and cramping while using Norplant.

What are the disadvantages?

Norplant does not protect you from sexually transmitted infections, including HIV. You may have more irregular bleeding and spotting during the first year after Norplant is inserted, or you may lose your period completely.

Some women complain of headaches, weight gain, depression, breast tenderness, and acne while using Norplant.

A minor surgical procedure is required to remove Norplant capsules.

How does this method affect your sexuality?

You don't have to worry about pregnancy, and sex can be spontaneous. Norplant, however, is a progestin and may decrease your desire and enjoyment of sex. And if you are having irregular bleeding, headaches, bloating, or other annoying side effects you can expect your desire for sex to plummet.

NuvaRing

NuvaRing is a soft, flexible, plastic ring containing estrogen and progestin hormones.

How does it work?
The ring releases a small amount of hormone daily to prevent ovulation.

How effective is it?
NuvaRing is very effective and has a failure rate of 1–2 percent.

How do you use it?
You insert the ring into your vagina and leave it there for three weeks. After three weeks, you remove the ring, wait one week, and then replace it with a new ring.

What are the advantages?
It is easy to use, effective, and easily reversible.

What are the disadvantages?
You must feel comfortable placing the ring in your vagina every month. The ring comes in only one size, so some women may find that the ring does not fit well. You or your partner may feel the ring during intercourse. The risks of complications with the ring are similar to those of the birth control pill, and smoking further increases those risks.

How does this method affect your sexuality?
The ring provides one month of protection so sex can be more spontaneous. The high effectiveness rate makes it easier to relax and enjoy sex without fear of pregnancy.

OrthoEvra
Also known as "the patch." It is a small, thin patch that is placed on your skin one day a week for three weeks out of each month. It slowly and continuously releases the same hormones, estrogen and progestin, that are present in birth control pills. Like the birth control pill, the patch is highly effective, and the risks are similar. The patch is not as effective in preventing pregnancy if you weigh more than 198 pounds.

Rhythm (Fertility Awareness, Natural Family Planning)

Fertility awareness is a method of birth control based on a calculation of your fertile period to prevent pregnancy.

How does it work?

You can predict when you are most likely to ovulate by measuring your temperature, checking your mucus, and/or counting the days of your cycle. You must abstain from intercourse or use another method of birth control during the days you are most fertile and most likely to get pregnant.

How effective is it?

If your periods are predictable and regular and you follow the rules perfectly, the chances of pregnancy are low—between 1 and 9 percent. However, the typical user of the rhythm method has a risk of pregnancy of 25 percent in the first year of use.

How do you use it?

There are three methods that can be used separately or together to determine your fertile days.

Calendar Method

- Record the first day of your period for six consecutive months before using the calendar method.

- Count the number of days in each cycle.

- Count from the first day of your period to the day prior to your next period.

- To find your earliest fertile day, take the number of days in your shortest cycle and subtract 18.

- To find your latest fertile day, take the number of days in your longest cycle and subtract 11.

⚚ You must abstain from sex or use another method of birth control during your fertile days (from the earliest fertile day to the latest fertile day).

Cervical Mucus Method

You can predict your fertile time by checking your mucus daily. Just before and at the time of ovulation, your mucus is thin, clear, and slippery. After ovulation, the mucus is thick and opaque. It is best to observe the changes in mucus for several months to learn your cycle.

Basal-Body-Temperature Method

You must take your temperature every morning before getting out of bed. After ovulation, your temperature rises between 0.4 and 0.8 degrees and remains up until your next period. You are safe to have sex three days after it is clear by your temperature that you have ovulated.

What are the advantages?

It is easy to use and has no side effects.

What are the disadvantages?

Natural family planning is effective only if you have regular, predictable periods. If you are peri-menopausal, postpartum, breast feeding, or have not established regular periods after using oral contraceptives, implants, or Depo-provera, your periods may not be predictable, and you should not use the rhythm method for contraception.

How does this method affect your sexuality?

Because you must be constantly aware of your fertility, the spontaneity of sex may be hampered. You may be forced to abstain from sex for many days during the month.

Spermicide

Spermicides are chemicals that are placed in your vagina before intercourse to kill sperm.

How does it work?

Spermicides prevent pregnancy by killing sperm before they can reach your uterus.

How effective is it?

The pregnancy rate during the first year of use varies from 6 to 26 percent. If you are young or having sex more than three times a week, your chances of getting pregnant may be higher.

How do you use it?

Spermicides can be purchased over the counter. You can choose a spermicidal cream, gel, foam, film, suppository, or tablet. Spermicide should be inserted high in your vagina near your cervix no less than 15 minutes and no more than 1 hour before having intercourse. If more than 1 hour passes before you have intercourse, or if you have sex more than once, you will need to insert more spermicide before intercourse.

What are the advantages?

Spermicides are easy to use, inexpensive, available in your local pharmacy, and they may decrease your risk of gonorrhea and chlamydia.

What are the disadvantages?

It is not clear what effect spermicides have on the virus that causes AIDS, and some studies have suggested that your risks of getting HIV may increase when using spermicides. Some women have more urinary tract and vaginal infections. Spermicides have a high failure rate.

How does this method affect your sexuality?

Spontaneity is lost since you must interrupt sex to insert the spermicide. Since the risks of pregnancy may be relatively high, fear of pregnancy may interfere with your desire and enjoyment of sex.

Female Sterilization: Tying Your Tubes

Female sterilization is a surgical procedure to block your fallopian tubes and permanently prevent pregnancy.

How does it work?

Your fallopian tubes carry your eggs from your ovary to your uterus. Female sterilization procedures interrupt your fallopian tubes so sperm cannot meet your egg.

How effective is it?

Female sterilization is a very effective method of contraception. The risks of pregnancy are usually less than 1 percent.

How do you use it?

Your doctor will perform a surgical procedure to burn, cut, tie, or clip your fallopian tubes.

What are the advantages?

Female sterilization is very effective and provides permanent protection against pregnancy.

What are the disadvantages?

Female sterilization should be considered a permanent method of contraception. It is not a good method for young women who may desire to have children later.

There is a small risk of serious injury from the female sterilization procedure, and a few women have pelvic pain, pain with their periods, pain with intercourse, and ovarian cysts after sterilization.

How does this method affect your sexuality?

You may have a marked increase in your desire and enjoyment of sex when the fear of pregnancy is permanently lifted. Some women have pain with sex during the first few months after the procedure. Changing your position during sex so that penetration is not as deep may be helpful, but be sure to talk to your doctor.

Male Sterilization (Vasectomy)

Vasectomy is a minor surgical procedure to block the tube that carries sperm.

When Contraception Fails

Aside from total abstinence, no method of contraception is 100 percent effective, and sometimes unintended pregnancies do occur. The decision to continue or end a pregnancy may not be an easy one and should not be made in haste. Carefully consider all of your options and do not hesitate to seek professional advice from your doctor, therapist, or Planned Parenthood. In the end, the decision is yours.

Pregnancy Termination

There are several options available for pregnancy termination in the United States today.

Vacuum aspiration: A surgical procedure that can be done in your doctor's office or a hospital. A machine that creates suction is used to remove the contents of your uterus under local anesthesia.

Mifepristone (RU 486): This drug has been available in Europe for over a decade and has been approved for use in the United States after years of debate and controversy. It is effective if no more than seven weeks have passed since the first day of your last menstrual period.

Methotrexate and misoprostol: Methotrexate is a medication that is given by injection. Several days later, a second drug, misoprostol, is placed in your vagina, causing your uterus to empty.

Having the Baby

If you make the decision to continue the pregnancy and have a baby, start taking prenatal vitamins containing folic acid as soon as you miss your

continued

period. You should also schedule an appointment with a doctor or midwife. Early and continuous prenatal care is important to assure both a healthy baby and a healthy mom.

How does it work?

The *vas deferens,* the tube that carries sperm from the testicle to be mixed with semen, is cut. Sperm are not released and thus cannot meet your egg.

How effective is it?

The risk of pregnancy after your partner has a vasectomy is very low, about 0.1 percent.

How do you use it?

Your partner's doctor will perform the procedure in his/her office or in the ambulatory unit of a hospital. You must use another method of birth control until his doctor finds that there are no more sperm in his ejaculate. Commonly, it may take 20 ejaculations before his semen is clear of sperm.

What are the advantages?

Vasectomy is a simple procedure that allows the male to participate in birth control. It is considered a permanent procedure, though in some cases it can be reversed.

What are the disadvantages?

Vasectomy does not prevent the spread of sexually transmitted infections.

How does this method affect your sexuality?

It's wonderful to have the responsibility of birth control lifted, and most women find that they have increased desire and enjoyment of sex.

Chapter 15

In Control: Safer Sex

Maybe you've only known him for a night or perhaps you've been together for a while. What matters is that for this moment he is exactly what you want. As you find yourself entangled in the sheets, the back of the car, or wherever this rendevous is taking place, you realize that there is a problem. Neither of you has a condom. What do you do?

- Think to yourself, "He's too cute and successful to have an STI."

- Think to yourself, "It feels too good to stop now!"

- Think to yourself, "I'll think about it tomorrow."

- Ask him if he has a disease and when he says "no" decide to continue full steam ahead.

- Stop and wait until you have a condom.

The answer may seem obvious to you now, but many of us would find ourselves caught up in the heat of the moment and unable to think clearly. That's why the time to think about sexually transmitted infections is before you find yourself in a similar situation. Knowing what infections exist and how to protect yourself is necessary to fully enjoy the pleasures of sexual intimacy.

Sexually transmitted infections are very common. Some would say that they are occurring in epidemic proportions. And it is a myth that only "bad" women get them. STIs don't discriminate, and anyone can catch one. You need only have intimate contact with one individual to become infected, and it is a misconception that you need to have intercourse to get an STI. Infections can be transmitted through oral, anal, or vaginal sex, but you can also get some infections simply by having skin-to-skin contact with an infected person.

STIs are more easily transmitted to women than men and, if left untreated, cause us more harm. They can lead to serious and permanent damage to your pelvis, which can result in chronic pelvic pain, infertility, pain with sex, cervical cancer, vaginal cancer, anal cancer, vulvar cancer, miscarriages, ectopic pregnancies, or even death. However, most STIs can be treated and cured, and the earlier you are treated the better.

With so much potentially at risk, it is imperative that you take charge of your sexual health. This includes:

- Be sure to request testing for all STIs yearly or each time you change sexual partners. Not all gynecologists test routinely for STIs so be sure to ask. Many STIs are asymptomatic, which is why often the only way to know you have one is to be tested.

- Between visits to your doctor, practice self-exam at home. Using a mirror in a well-lit room, inspect your vulva, vaginal opening, and anus monthly. Look for bumps, sores, ulcers, areas of redness or swelling, or unusual discharge. Report any unusual findings to your doctor immediately.

- **Be sure to see your doctor if your partner complains of a problem or you have unprotected sex.**

Talking to Your Partner About Safer Sex

Most people who pass on STIs are not even aware that they have an infection. That means that the only way to completely protect yourself from infection is to abstain from sexual contact. It is also possible to have mind-blowing sex that is both safe and healthy. Begin by talking openly and frankly to your partner about safer sex prior to getting into bed. Don't wait until you are in the throes of passion to begin to talk because you may find your judgment clouded by the emotions and good feelings that you are experiencing. It can be difficult and embarrassing to talk freely about sex, but oh so necessary for your health. Ask directly about your partner's history of sexually transmitted infections and let him know that you have decided to practice safer sex every time you have sex. Assume that he has an infection until proven otherwise and practice safer sex. Life is too precious and much too short to take risks.

Reducing Your Risks of an STI

- Limit yourself to mutually monogamous relationships with partners that are not infected.

- Always use condoms for vaginal, anal, and oral sex and for covering sex toys; use dental dams or plastic wrap for oral stimulation of the vulva or anus; and use latex gloves to cover broken skin when manually stimulating your partner.

- Avoid high-risk sexual practices until you and your partner have been tested for STIs and, if necessary, treated for any infections. High-risk activities include anal intercourse and vaginal intercourse. Practices such as hugging, cuddling, massage, mutual masturbation, sharing fantasies, and erotica can be satisfying and are low-risk activities.

- Be careful when mixing alcohol and sex. Alcohol can cloud your judgment and increase the chances that you will make a bad decision.

ꙮ Limit your number of sexual partners. The more partners you
have, the greater your chances of getting an STI.

ꙮ You and your partner should get tested for sexually transmitted
infections prior to having sex. Repeat the tests six months later.
If you have both been monogamous and are both negative for
STIs, you can have sex without a condom.

ꙮ Take the time to examine your male partner before having sex.

Examining Your Male Partner

Before you turn off the lights, take the time to examine your male partner
for signs of a sexually transmitted infection. You may be embarrassed, but
remember that as an adult you owe it to yourself and your partner—
present and future—to be responsible. With the right attitude, you can
turn this into another part of your foreplay.

Start your inspection at the top of his pubic hair. Look for bumps, blisters, ulcers, sores, rashes, and red areas among the pubic hair. Continue by
moving along the entire shaft of his penis, including the underside. Don't
forget to look at the head; pull back the foreskin if he is not circumcised,
noting any discharge that might be expressed. A yellow or milky-white discharge may be a sign of gonorrhea or chlamydia. Hold his penis firmly but
gently in your hand and slide it from the base of his penis to the head with
a milking motion. Next examine the front and the underside of his scrotum, making a mental note of all bumps and sores. Finally, end with an inspection of the skin surrounding his anus.

To turn the examination into something much sexier, use your hands to
massage warm oil as you carefully inspect his genitals. You can do an expert inspection as he moans in pleasure. Of course, if you find a suspicious lesion, you should not have sex, even with a condom, until he has
seen a doctor. A condom may not protect you completely if he has an active infection.

The vinegar test can also be used for more extensive examination of
your partner for sexually transmitted infections. It will require his cooper-
ation, but if you are suspicious you should demand it.

Take a number of gauze pads and soak them in white vinegar. Wrap his penis and scrotum loosely with the wet gauze and allow it to remain in place for 5 minutes. Remove the gauze and look for areas of skin on or near his penis and scrotum that have turned white. These areas may represent an infection with the human papilloma virus that causes genital warts. It is also possible that the areas do not represent an infection but a visit to a doctor is in order before having sex. Do not attempt this test if your partner has open sores or irritated, broken skin since the vinegar will burn. Keep in mind that your partner may have an STI and not have any symptoms or signs of an infection. You should practice safer sex until you are certain that your partner has been adequately tested for sexually transmitted infections.

You're probably saying to yourself, "How can I possibly risk insulting him by asking to marinate his penis in vinegar?" Well, I ask you, "Is your sexual health and your life worth risking to protect his feelings?" You might also let him know that some sexually transmitted infections, if not treated, increase his risks of cancer of the penis, the treatment of which may include removing his penis.

The Lowdown on Latex and Other Safer Sex Aids

Male Condoms

The gold standard of safer sex is the use of latex condoms. Though not completely protective against all STIs, condoms can significantly reduce the chances that you will become infected if used correctly and every time you have vaginal intercourse, anal sex, or oral sex.

Condoms made of latex, polyurethane, and a new synthetic called Tactylon have been shown to be effective against STIs. Condoms will not protect you, however, if your partner has an infectious lesion or sore that is not covered by the condom, such as herpes sores or warts on the base of his penis or scrotum. The natural-skin condoms may protect you from pregnancy but do not protect you from sexually transmitted infections. And condoms sold as novelties do not protect you from sexually transmitted infections or pregnancy.

How to Put On a Condom

To be effective against STIs and pregnancy, a condom must be put on before there is any contact between his penis and your genitals. If you feel uncomfortable handling them, practice rolling on a condom using a cucumber or zucchini to make it easier when you are in the throes of passion. And remember to only use condoms that have been properly stored in a cool, dry place and that have not passed the expiration date printed on the package.

To use one, carefully open the package, making sure to keep long fingernails and teeth from damaging the condom. Inspect the condom to see if it is dry, sticky, or brittle, in which case it should be discarded. Unroll the condom a little bit and place a few drops of water-based lubricant inside the tip to increase his sensitivity and pleasure. Next place the condom over the head of his penis, slowly unrolling it down the shaft. If he is not circumcised, pull his foreskin back as you roll. Make sure that you leave a little bit of space at the top of the condom to catch his sperm. Some condoms have a special reservoir tip designed for this purpose. Apply water-based lubricant to the outside of the condom and inside your vagina or anus to prevent breakage and make sex more pleasurable for you and your partner.

As soon as he ejaculates, his penis must be withdrawn. If you wait, his penis may become soft and the condom can slip off, releasing semen. As he withdraws his penis, hold the condom at the base of his penis. Discard the condom immediately following sex. If you have intercourse again, a new condom must be used.

NOTE: *If the condom breaks while you are having intercourse, stop and place contraceptive foam or cream in your vagina. Use a new condom to continue intercourse.*

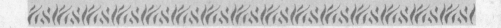

Let's be frank, we'd all prefer to have sex without a condom. The feel of nice warm skin is preferable to that of latex or plastic, even if the sheath is ultrathin. But is it really worth the chance of a serious infection or the loss of your life for a few minutes of naked pleasure? The answer is obvious.

Female Condoms

The Reality female condom is highly effective in protecting you from sexually transmitted infections. It is made of polyurethane and can be used if you are allergic to latex. Because it covers your vagina and most of your vulva, it protects you from most STIs, including herpes and genital warts, better than the male condom. The female condom also gives you control over your sexual health, especially if your partner does not want to wear a condom. Some men and women find the female condom to be more stimulating than the male condom.

Dental Dams and Plastic Wrap

A dental dam is a small latex square, traditionally used by dentists, that can be placed over the vulva or anus of your partner during oral sex. They come in different sizes and flavors and can be used only once. The square must be held in place to prevent exposure to vaginal or anal secretions or lesions. To increase the pleasure of your partner, place water-based lubricant on your partner's genitals or on the side of the dam that is touching his or her skin. Glyde dams are thinner than traditional dental dams and are approved by the Federal Drug Administration.

Plastic wrap (straight from the supermarket shelf) is an alternative barrier that can be placed over the vulva and anus of your partner during oral sex. Because plastic wrap is thinner than dental dams, the sensations may be stronger.

Spermicides, Diaphragms, Cervical Caps, and Sponges

All barrier methods of contraception will decrease your risk of infection with gonorrhea and chlamydia. They have not been shown to protect against other STIs, including HIV infection.

Latex Gloves

It may not sound romantic to touch your lover with latex gloves, but if you are not sure whether your sex partner has a sexually transmitted infection, especially HIV, and you have tiny cuts, abrasions, ingrown nails, skin infections, or rashes on your hands, you need to protect yourself with gloves. Gloves will protect you from vaginal and rectal secretions that may carry sexually transmitted bacteria or viruses. Use lots of water-based lubricants to increase the pleasure of your partner.

STIs: What You Need to Know

Chancroid

Chancroid infection is caused by a bacterium, *Hemophilus ducreyi*. It is not common in the United States.

How is it transmitted?

Chancroid is transmitted when you have oral, vaginal, or anal sex with a person who is infected with the bacterium.

How is it diagnosed?

Approximately seven days after having sex with an infected partner, you may notice one or several painful ulcers on your vulva or the opening to your vagina. You may also notice tender, swollen glands (lymph nodes) in the space between your hips and mons. Your doctor will send a special culture to make the diagnosis.

How is it treated?

Chancroid is easily treated with antibiotics.

How does it affect my sexuality?

Your sexual partner(s) should be told that you have the infection and he (they) should be treated. There is no need to inform future sex partners once you have been treated.

Chlamydia

Chlamydia infection is caused by a bacterium, *Chlamydia trachomatis,* that usually infects your cervix or urethra. It is the most common sexually transmitted infection in the United States, with 3 million cases occurring annually. Chlamydia is known as the "silent" sexually transmitted infection because most women who have it do not have symptoms.

How is it transmitted?

Chlamydia infections are most commonly spread by vaginal intercourse. It is also possible to spread the bacterium through anal intercourse or oral sex and by sharing sex toys. Using a condom during anal, vaginal, and oral sex and when sharing sex toys will protect you from infection with chlamydia. Diaphragms, cervical caps, and contraceptive sponges also decrease your chances of infection.

How is it diagnosed?

The infection usually begins one to three weeks after having unprotected sex with someone infected with the bacterium, but most women do not have symptoms. So you can have it for many months without knowing that you are infected. Ten percent of women will notice a heavy, yellow discharge, bleeding after sex, bleeding between periods, fever, pelvic pain, pain with sex, or burning when urinating.

The diagnosis is made when your doctor performs a special culture for chlamydia. Many doctors, however, don't test routinely for chlamydia, so be sure to ask for a culture yearly or every time you change sexual partners.

How is it treated?

Chlamydia is easily treated with antibiotics. It is very important to take all of the medication that your doctor prescribes even if you are feeling better. A repeat culture should be done three weeks after you complete the treatment. Your most recent sexual partner and any sex partners that you have had intimate contact with in the previous two months must be notified and treated—even if he has no symptoms (a man will sometimes have a discharge from his penis and burning when he urinates but may have no symptoms at all). Do not have sex while you are being treated and not before you and your partner have had negative repeat cultures.

Early diagnosis and treatment are important; if left unchecked, chlamydia can cause a more severe pelvic infection called *pelvic inflammatory disease (PID)*. PID can damage your fallopian tubes and cause infertility or chronic pain in your pelvis.

How does it affect my sexuality?

Chlamydia is easily treated and cured when diagnosed early. There is no need to inform future sex partners once you have been successfully treated. Using a condom or other barrier during sex will protect you from reinfection.

Gonorrhea

Gonorrhea infection is caused by *Neisseria gonorrhea*, a bacterium that can infect your cervix, throat, rectum, and urethra.

How is it transmitted?

Gonorrhea is transmitted when you have vaginal, anal, or oral sex with an infected partner. The bacteria reside in the urethra of infected men and can be transferred in semen to your mouth, urethra, cervix, and anus during sex. Male and female condoms, diaphragms, cervical caps, and sponges decrease your risk of infection with gonorrhea.

How is it diagnosed?

Most women with gonorrhea do not have symptoms. Those who do have symptoms will notice a yellow vaginal discharge, burning and soreness of the vulva, burning when urinating, pain or bleeding during sex, sore throat, or bleeding between periods beginning around 10 days after having contact with an infected partner. Your doctor can make the diagnosis by taking a culture of your cervix, throat, and/or anus. Because some doctors don't routinely culture every patient for gonorrhea, you should request a culture for gonorrhea during your yearly pelvic exam and after starting a new sexual relationship. You should also ask for a culture if your partner complains of a discharge from his penis or burning when he urinates.

How is it treated?

Gonorrhea infections are easily treated with antibiotics. Your doctor may treat you with an injection, pills, or a combination of the two. Because chlamydia usually resides with gonorrhea, you should be treated for both infections at the same time. Your last sexual partner and all sexual partners in the 60 days prior to being diagnosed must be informed and treated. Do not have sex until you and your partner have been treated and your follow-up cultures show that you are no longer infected with gonorrhea.

Left untreated, gonorrhea can cause pelvic inflammatory disease, damage to your fallopian tubes, ectopic pregnancy, infertility, chronic pelvic pain, and pain with sex.

How does it affect my sexuality?

Gonorrhea is easily treated and cured when diagnosed early. There is no need to inform your future sex partners of your past history of gonorrhea once you have been successfully treated. Taking charge of your sexuality and practicing safer sex will make it easier for you to resume a normal, healthy sex life.

Hepatitis B

Hepatitis B infection is caused by the hepatitis B virus (HBV) which can infect and damage your liver.

How is it transmitted?

This virus can be transmitted in blood, saliva, semen, and vaginal secretions and may be spread through unprotected oral, vaginal, or anal intercourse. Using a condom every time you have sex can protect you from infection with hepatitis B virus. HBV can also be transmitted through intravenous drug use and blood transfusions.

How is it diagnosed?

Many people with hepatitis have no symptoms. Those who do have symptoms may experience decreased appetite, weight loss, indigestion, nausea, vomiting, and fatigue. Your doctor can make the diagnosis by performing a blood test for hepatitis B.

How is it treated?

There is no treatment for hepatitis B infection; however, your immune system will most likely fight the infection successfully. All sex partners should be informed that you have the virus and should be tested. I recommend that all sexually active women get the vaccination for hepatitis B to protect them from possible infection.

How does it affect my sexuality?

A small number of women infected with the virus will become chronic carriers of the virus and can transmit it to their sex partners. Your doctor can do tests to find out if you are at risk of transmitting the virus to others. If you are found to be a carrier of hepatitis B, your future sex partners must be informed before having sex.

Hepatitis C

Hepatitis C is similar to hepatitis B. Although hepatitis C can be sexually transmitted, most cases result from IV drug use. If you are sexually active and have multiple sex partners or if your partner uses IV drugs, you should ask your doctor to test you for hepatitis C infection. Using condoms can decrease your risks of getting hepatitis C infection.

Herpes

Herpes is a common sexually transmitted infection caused by the herpes virus (HSV). One in five American adults have been infected with genital herpes. Two types of herpes virus can cause infection of your genitals: herpes virus type 1 and herpes virus type 2. Herpes type 1 most commonly infects your mouth but can be transmitted to your genitals through oral sex. You can also infect your own genitals by touching them after touching a fresh cold sore on your lip. Herpes type 2 more commonly affects the genitals, but it can also be transmitted to your mouth during oral sex. Genital infections with herpes type 1 tend to be milder and don't recur as often as infections with type 2.

How is it transmitted?

Herpes is transmitted when you have close, intimate contact with the active herpes lesions of an infected partner. You don't have to have intercourse to become infected with genital herpes, and a condom may not protect you completely from infection: If your partner has a lesion on his scrotum, anus, or any area that is not covered by the condom, you can become infected.

How is it diagnosed?

Many women with herpes have no symptoms and are not aware that they are infected. If you do have symptoms, you may notice blisters or ulcers on your vulva or vagina. You may have many sores or one tiny spot the size of a pinhead, and they may last for a few days to a few weeks. The lesions may be very painful or may itch.

The best way for your doctor to diagnose herpes is to do a special culture for the herpes virus. The culture is most accurate if done when you have a fresh blister or ulcer. The blood test for herpes can be misleading because most of us have had cold sores and are positive for past herpes type 1 virus infection. Most blood tests can't distinguish between infections caused by herpes type 1 and type 2.

How is it treated?

There is no cure for genital herpes infection. However, there are medications that decrease the duration of an active outbreak and make you feel better faster. Your doctor may prescribe pills that are taken 2 to 5 times a day for 5 to 10 days. With or without treatment, the lesions caused by herpes will go away but the virus will remain in your body. It travels up nerves to the nerve roots, where it waits quietly. The virus can travel back down the nerve at a later time and cause a recurrence of the herpes infection. No one knows what causes the virus to reemerge. Everyone's experience of herpes is different. You may have many frequent recurrences or you may never have another genital lesion after the first episode. Many women have noticed that emotional or physical stress causes more frequent herpes outbreaks. Therefore, I recommend a healthy diet, exercise, and a lifestyle in which stress reduction is a priority.

Antiviral medication should be started as soon as you notice the onset of a herpes outbreak. If you have frequent outbreaks (six or more episodes per year) your doctor may recommend that you take antiviral medication every day for up to one year to reduce the number of outbreaks. As time passes, you will probably notice that you get fewer and milder outbreaks.

How does it affect my sexuality?

Getting a diagnosis of herpes infection can be alarming. You may experience anger, confusion, disbelief, and fear, and your desire for sex may immediately take a nosedive. Fear that you might transmit the virus to others may prevent you from fully enjoying sex. Learn as much as you can about herpes and how your body responds to the infection so that you can have herpes and still have a fantastic sex life.

The rules are simple and easy to follow once you get to know your herpes. When you have an active lesion, you should not have sex, not even with a condom. As you become more familiar with how your body responds to the infection, you may notice that you have symptoms such as tingling, itching, or burning in the area where your herpes sores usually appear hours or days in advance of an actual lesion. You can transmit the virus during this time and should not have sex—even with a condom. When there are no active lesions, you can have sex. Though you can transmit the virus when you have no symptoms, the chances are very small. Using a condom will decrease the chance that you will transmit the infection to your partner.

Discuss your herpes infection before any sexual activity with a new partner. Be honest and informative. Herpes is so common that it is highly unlikely that a new partner will be shocked or overly concerned about your history of herpes. If he leaves because of your honest disclosure, he probably wasn't worth your emotional investment anyway.

Every woman wants to know where she got it from. Unfortunately, unless you have had only one sex partner, it is impossible to tell. The virus can lurk undetected for years before a lesion appears. In my practice, I have seen women who developed their first herpes lesion after 20 years of celibacy.

Human Immunodeficiency Virus (HIV)

HIV has single-handedly changed the sexual practices of millions of people. HIV infection is caused by the human immunodeficiency virus, which attacks your immune system and prevents it from protecting you against infections. HIV eventually causes AIDS, a fatal disease.

How is it transmitted?

The HIV virus can be found in saliva, blood, semen, vaginal secretions, and breast milk. The virus can be transmitted through blood transfusions, intravenous drug use, breast feeding, and sexual activities. The risk of transmission is highest with anal intercourse, but the virus can also be transmitted through vaginal intercourse, oral sex—giving and receiving oral sex have risks—and sharing sex toys. The risks with kissing and mutual masturbation are much lower.

Though not 100 percent effective, using a latex or polyurethane condom every time you have sex will decrease your risks of becoming infected with HIV. Your risks of contracting HIV are increased if you have another sexually transmitted infection.

How is it diagnosed?

The diagnosis is made by blood tests to detect the antibody to HIV. It may take up to six months for the antibody test to become positive after you have been exposed to the virus. Most people in the early phases of HIV infection have no symptoms; others will notice symptoms that include fever, severe fatigue, swollen lymph nodes, and a skin rash in the first few weeks of infection with HIV. Late signs of HIV include fever, weight loss, cough, and diarrhea. If you are starting a relationship with a new partner, you should both be tested for HIV. Once you are both found to be negative, you should use condoms and be monogamous. After six months have passed, the test should be repeated to be certain that neither of you has the virus. If you both remain negative and are still monogamous, it is safe to have sex without a condom.

How is it treated?

There is no cure for HIV infection, and most people infected with HIV will develop AIDS within 17 years of diagnosis. There are antiviral medications now available that may be effective in slowing the progress from HIV infection to the development of AIDS. All sex partners must be notified of your HIV status, and they must be tested.

How does it affect my sexuality?

A diagnosis of HIV infection can be devastating. Your desire for sex, arousal, and ability to respond sexually may all be hampered by your diagnosis. However, it is possible to have a satisfying sex life after HIV. You will need to learn new low-risk ways to express yourself sexually, and practicing safer sex is a must. All future sex partners must be informed of your infection prior to any intimate contact. Talk to a counselor or join support groups to learn effective methods for maintaining a healthy life and sexuality with HIV.

Human Papilloma Virus (HPV)

Human papilloma virus is the virus that causes *genital warts*. HPV is the most common sexually transmitted viral infection in the United States; some researchers estimate that more than 40 percent of sexually active women have been exposed to the virus, and perhaps as many as 90 percent will be exposed during their lifetime. There are many different types of human papilloma virus, and HPV may infect your vulva, vagina, anus, or cervix. Some low-risk types cause common benign warts whereas other, high-risk types have been associated with cancer of the vulva, vagina, cervix, or anus.

How is it transmitted?

HPV is transmitted when you have skin-to-skin contact with a person infected with HPV. It is not necessary to have vaginal intercourse to become infected. If your partner has warts on his penis, scrotum, or anus, and those warts touch your genital area, you may become infected. Using a condom every time you have sex will decrease your chances of being exposed to HPV but is not a guarantee. You may still be exposed to the virus if he has lesions on parts of his genitals that are not covered by the condom. Examining his genitals for warts can further decrease the chances that you will become infected, though many men do not have any visible symptoms.

How is it diagnosed?

Many women and men who have the human papilloma virus have no symptoms and are not aware that they are infected. For those who do have symptoms, infection with HPV may cause bumps that are flesh-colored, grayish, or slightly darker than their skin. Some may look like tiny cauliflowers and some may be flat; they may itch or burn. You may have no symptoms and discover the warts only during self-examination. If you have the typical lesions on your vulva, vaginal opening, or near your anus, the diagnosis may be obvious. Still, your doctor may suggest a biopsy to be certain of the diagnosis.

HPV infection may also cause your pap smear to be abnormal. Your doctor may recommend special tests to make the diagnosis. A *colposcope* (a microscope on a stick) may be used in the office to magnify your cervix, and a biopsy may be performed.

How is it treated?

There is no cure for HPV infection. However, recent studies have shown that, over time, your immune system may totally clear the virus from your body. Warts that are obvious should be treated—with laser, freezing, cutting, or burning with creams or acids—to decrease the chances of transmitting the virus to a partner. You may need to be treated several times before the warts go away. Treating the obvious lesions, however, may not get rid of the virus. The virus may still lurk in the skin surrounding the wart and warts may recur later.

For some women HPV will cause an abnormal pap smear. If you are infected with a low-risk type of HPV, your doctor may decide to watch and wait for a year before treating you. Infections with these low-risk types of HPV will spontaneously disappear in 80 percent of infected women within a year. If your abnormality is more severe or caused by a type of HPV that has been associated with cervical cancer, you may need to be treated with cryotherapy, laser, or a large biopsy. Once you have been diagnosed with HPV, you should get a repeat pap smear every 6–12 months.

How does it affect my sexuality?

Your sex partner(s) should be examined and any warts should be treated. You may become angry with your sex partner for exposing you to the virus, but unless he is the only person you have ever had intimate contact with, it is impossible to determine with absolute certainty that he is the person who gave you the infection. Some women can be infected with the virus for years before noticing a lesion or showing a change in their pap smear.

Because so many people have the human papilloma virus, chances are good that your future sex partner has also been exposed in the past. I suggest that you tell future sex partners that you have been exposed to the virus and treated before you have sex. Let him know that the chances of transmitting the virus when you don't have a lesion are small. Do not have sex when you have an obvious lesion, and use condoms at other times to decrease the chance that you may pass the virus to your sex partner.

Keep in mind that HPV infection is very common. You are not alone and have not done anything wrong. There is no reason to feel guilt or shame. It only takes one exposure to the virus to become infected.

Molluscum Contagiosum

Molluscum contagiosum is a skin infection caused by a virus that may be sexually transmitted in adults. The infection begins three to six weeks after exposure.

How is it transmitted?

The virus is transmitted when you have close, intimate skin-to-skin contact with a person infected with molluscum contagiosum. It can also be transmitted through nonsexual contact with an infected person or through sharing towels.

How is it diagnosed?

Infection with molluscum contagiosum causes painless, small, smooth, dome-shaped shiny bumps on your vulva and inner thighs. The bumps sometimes have a dimple in the center. Your doctor can usually make the diagnosis by examining you, though a biopsy may be done to make sure the diagnosis is correct.

How is it treated?

The infection may disappear spontaneously, but persistent infections can be treated with cryotherapy (freezing), scraping, or burning with chemicals. Your sexual partners should also be examined and treated.

How does it affect my sexuality?

Molluscum contagiosum infection does not cause any complications and has no effect on your sexuality. There is no need to inform future sex partners of a past infection with molluscum contagiosum.

Pubic Lice

Pubic lice, or "crabs," are parasites that infect your vulva.

How is it transmitted?

Pubic lice are transmitted when you have close, intimate contact with an infected partner. You can also pick up the bugs when you share the bed linens, towels, and clothing of an infected person.

How is it diagnosed?

The lice live in your pubic hair and cause intense itching. Close inspection by your doctor will reveal the lice.

How is it treated?

Lice are easily killed by using Kwell, Rid, or Triple X shampoo. Only one dose is necessary. All underwear, towels, and bed linens should be washed in hot water to kill any lice or eggs before reuse, and your sexual partner should be treated.

How does it affect my sexuality?

Lice infection has no effect on your sexuality.

Syphilis

Syphilis is a very old disease that, though less common today, continues to rear its ugly head. Syphilis is caused by a tiny spiral-shaped organism called *Treponema pallidum*.

How is it transmitted?

Syphilis is transmitted through direct contact with an infected sore or ulcer on your external genitals, vagina, anus, lips, mouth, or rectum. A pregnant woman can pass it to her baby.

How is it diagnosed?

The first sign of syphilis may be an ulcer or sore on your vulva, vagina, or cervix that appears two to four weeks after exposure to an infected partner. The ulcer usually does not hurt or itch. In fact, you may not even be aware that it is present. The diagnosis is usually made by a blood test.

How is it treated?

Early syphilis is treated with an injection of penicillin (or another antibiotic if you are allergic to penicillin). Left untreated, syphilis may cause extensive damage to your brain, heart, joints, and eyes. Your sexual partners must be informed and treated.

How does it affect my sexuality?

You may feel confused and frightened when you find out that you have syphilis, but remember that it is fully treatable with antibiotics. There is no need to inform future sex partners of a past infection with syphilis.

Trichomoniasis

Trichomoniasis (trich) is caused by a small parasite, *Trichomonas vaginalis*. Though it is generally considered a sexually transmitted infection, women who have never been sexually active have been diagnosed with the infection.

How is it transmitted?

Most cases of trich infection are transmitted through vaginal intercourse.

How is it diagnosed?

Trichomoniasis typically produces a heavy, frothy, yellow or greenish discharge that may have a foul odor and cause severe itching or irritation of your vulva and vagina. Your doctor can make the diagnosis by looking at a drop of your vaginal discharge under a microscope or by sending a specimen for culture to the lab.

How is it treated?

Trichomoniasis is treated with the antibiotic metronidazole in a single dose or over the course of seven days. Your sex partner should be treated at the same time. Most men with trichomoniasis infection do not have symptoms. You should delay intercourse until you and your partner have been successfully treated to prevent reinfection.

How does it affect my sexuality?

Trichomoniasis is easily treated and does not affect your sexuality.

If you suspect that you have a sexually transmitted infection, you may feel ashamed, afraid, and confused. Do not be embarrassed to discuss your concerns with your doctor. Sexually transmitted infections are very common, and most can be completely treated with medication. Early diagnosis and treatment are key to your future health and happiness.

Part IV

Sex
for Life

Chapter 16

Sex and Pregnancy

Almost every newly pregnant couple comes to me with the same question, and my answer never changes: "Yes, you can continue to have sex. It is perfectly safe and won't hurt your baby. In fact, if you both desire it, some studies suggest that satisfying sex is good for pregnancy."

Your sex life doesn't have to end with pregnancy. But it may change. During pregnancy, levels of different hormones fluctuate—sometimes wildly—which, in turn, can cause your sexual desire to fluctuate, too. As your body and your baby grow, you may also begin to feel differently about yourself and your body, which can also affect the way you feel about sex. There really is no norm for sexual behavior; every woman and every couple is different.

The most important things to remember are to pay close attention to the changes in your body and to acknowledge and honor your emotions. Communicating with your partner during pregnancy is, of course, critical. Talk about how you are feeling, physically and emotionally, and be sure to encourage him to talk about his feelings as well. That will help ensure that your sexual relations are as healthy as you and your baby.

How You May Be Feeling About Sex

For some women, pregnancy is a time of increased arousal. Once your pregnancy hormones kick in, you may be feeling very interested in having sex. Depending on the stage of pregnancy, the changes in your body may make you feel very sexy and erotic. Changes in your body may even make orgasms more intense. You may love your developing body, your larger breasts and brand-new curves. The freedom of not having to worry about birth control may also add to the excitement. Having sex with your partner, especially if the sight of your pregnant body excites him, may be highly satisfying during this time and can give the two of you a lovely opportunity to strengthen your ties and share intimacy and pleasure before your new baby arrives.

Other women react differently to their hormonal fluctuations and their changing bodies. You may not feel like having sex often or at all. It may be too uncomfortable, most likely during the first and last trimesters, or you may have trouble reaching a climax. You may not like how your body looks and feels, and even though people—your partner included—may be telling you how beautiful you are, you may not be feeling it. You may simply feel fat and overburdened by the growing life inside of you. You may be worried and stressed out, especially if you're pregnant with your first child and aren't entirely sure what to expect.

You and your partner may worry that sex may hurt the baby. But if you feel like making love, and your pregnancy is not high risk, you can keep doing it safely until your water breaks. Sex won't hurt your baby, and having an orgasm won't throw you into labor or trigger a miscarriage. However, if you have a history of premature labor or repeated miscarriage, you may be advised to forgo sexual relations. Your husband's penis won't harm your baby, and sperm inside of you won't cause an infection. Finally, the baby doesn't know that you're having sex. You may feel increased movement of

Who Should Say No to Sex

Some women have medical conditions that may make having sex or orgasm (even through masturbation) risky during pregnancy. Be sure to talk to your health-care provider about any of the conditions below.

You may not be able to have sex if:

- You are considered "high risk." In this case, your doctor may advise abstaining from sex during part or all of your pregnancy. Discuss with her whether intercourse or orgasm (or both) is not advised.

- You have vaginal bleeding.

- You have a history of miscarriages.

- You have dilation of your cervix. (Only your health-care provider will be able to determine this.)

- You have ruptured your membranes, which means that your water has broken.

- You've had premature labor in the past.

- You have *placenta previa,* which occurs when the placenta is located over the cervix. Intercourse could damage the placenta and cause severe bleeding.

- You have twins or more. Your health-care provider may advise you to abstain during the second half of your pregnancy.

- You have toxemia, or pregnancy-related high blood pressure.

the fetus after orgasm, but that's a normal result of small, harmless contractions of your uterus. Relax—your baby is safe and well protected.

Your Sexuality: A Trimester-by-Trimester Guide

Sexual feelings are different for each pregnant woman and may also vary from one stage of pregnancy to another. This is what you may experience during the different stages:

First Trimester: The Beginning of Your Pregnancy

During these first 12 weeks, many women experience intense physical symptoms that may affect how they feel sexually.

Physical Changes That May Affect Sexuality

One of the first signs of pregnancy is enlargement and increased tenderness of your breasts. While some women are proud of the increased size of their breasts and feel more erotic, having their breasts touched may also cause them discomfort. And if breast stimulation has been a major part of your sex play with your partner, you may feel less enthusiastic about sex. If so, ask him to be gentle, handle with care, or find other erogenous zones. You can also wear a bra (even a sexy one!) to bed to support your breasts and make you feel more comfortable. Experiment with positions that take pressure off your breasts.

Another early sign of pregnancy is nausea. For some women nausea starts in the morning and may continue for most or all of the day. When your stomach is turning it is difficult to even *think* of sex play. You can help curb nausea by eating small meals throughout the day, avoiding foods that make you feel sick, taking your prenatal vitamins with a small amount of food or at bedtime, and drinking some kinds of herbal tea.

In the early weeks of pregnancy, you may feel extremely tired. You may find it difficult to get out of bed in the morning and completely run out of steam by mid-afternoon. Fatigue can depress your desire for sex. When you can barely drag yourself to bed to sleep, you are unlikely to have the energy and stamina for sex. It helps to get plenty of rest during this period and also to vary the times you make love to coincide with your higher energy levels.

Soon after you become pregnant, blood flow to your pelvis increases, causing an engorged, swollen feeling in your pelvis. This sensation makes some women feel like they are in a constant state of arousal whereas others feel uncomfortable. This change may also affect your orgasms, making them easier or more difficult to achieve. Also, the increased blood flow combined with the enlarging uterus can make deep penetration uncomfortable. If so, ask your partner to go slow or find a position that's more pleasurable. You may also find that the use of water-based lubricants may make sex more comfortable. Remember that sex is more than intercourse. Hugging, cuddling, massage, kissing, and masturbation may be easier and just as enjoyable during this trimester.

Emotional Changes That May Affect Sexuality

At this point, your overriding fear may be miscarriage, especially if you've had one before. Though most miscarriages occur during the first trimester, having sex usually does not affect the risk. But if you do feel anxious, talk it over with your partner; you may feel more like being held and reassured than like making love.

Your moods may swing during this period of hormonal fluctuation, and this could affect how you feel about having sex. Many women say that they feel like crying all the time or seem to have little control of their emotions during early pregnancy. These mood swings may also cause you to feel hot and cold about sex. Fatigue and even anxiety over being newly pregnant can add to the problem and dampen your sex drive. Again, discuss these feelings with your partner.

Second Trimester: The Middle of Your Pregnancy

During the middle weeks of pregnancy, many women notice an easing of physical symptoms. Nausea often subsides, breast tenderness abates, and fatigue diminishes—you may be feeling great, even energetic. If you're also feeling sexy, these three months may be the best time for you to enjoy making love while you're expecting.

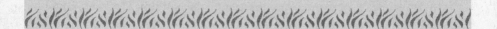

His Feelings

For some men, sex during pregnancy is incredibly hot, whereas for others it is a turn-off and even frightening. The important thing to remember is that just as your feelings may change during your pregnancy, his may too. The key is to communicate frequently and openly about how each of you is feeling and to try to avoid power struggles over sex.

He may be feeling turned on by your body. That's great as long as you are feeling sexual as well. Be clear about your own feelings and encourage him to do the same so that the two of you can maintain intimacy and stay connected throughout your pregnancy.

Perhaps he fears that he may injure you or the baby. He may not know that, as long as you are not considered high risk, sex is fine. Explain the facts to him and encourage him to seek further information. Reassure him that his touch is pleasurable and help him find a position that's comfortable for you.

He may not want sex as much as before. He may find the whole pregnancy thing—with its morning sickness and leaking breasts—unattractive and unsexy. He may have difficulty seeing you as a "lover" rather than a "mother." These feelings may make it difficult for him to get aroused and ejaculate. Though it's difficult and may make you feel bad, try not to take this personally. Every man is different, but it's important to honor each other's feelings—and fears.

He may feel that he is being replaced. Some men fear that the baby will take all of your attention. This may lead to anger and tension in the relationship, which can affect your sexual intimacy. Just as you need reassurance that you are still attractive to him and that everything will be okay once the baby comes, let him know that you still love him and that he's not going to be replaced by the new arrival.

Physical Changes That May Affect Sexuality

There is a further increase in blood flow to your genitals and pelvis during the second trimester. This may make it easier to achieve orgasm; orgasms may be more intense; and some women even have first orgasms during their second trimesters—or first multiple orgasms.

It is now extra important to experiment with various sexual positions to accommodate your growing belly. It might be more comfortable for you to be on top, or for the two of you to be side by side facing each other. You can also try "spooning" (both of you on your sides with him entering you or touching you from the rear); or you can crouch on your hands and knees while he enters you from the back; or both of you can sit with you on top. Use pillows to transform an awkward position into a pleasurable one.

Emotional Changes That May Affect Sexuality

Your overriding feeling during the second trimester may be relief from nausea, fatigue, and those sore, swollen breasts. As your symptoms abate— and your energy increases—you may feel like having sex, even a lot. Although your desire may increase during this period, it may still be less than it was before pregnancy. You should also try not to worry if you continue to feel your desire waning; this is normal, too.

During the second trimester, you will also begin to "show," and your weight gain and changing shape may make you feel unattractive. Communication is key, so mention these feelings to your partner. On the other hand, your new body may make you feel like a sexy, voluptuous goddess.

Third Trimester: The Last Leg of Your Pregnancy

During the final months of your pregnancy, your body will be getting quite large, and you may feel very unwieldy. The feeling of extreme fatigue will probably return, and you may have no desire to make love. A few women will find this trimester to be the sexiest of all.

Physical Changes That May Affect Sexuality

Just about every pregnant woman feels tired—if not exhausted—during the final trimester. In addition, sleep may be difficult, partly because it

Sexual Practices During Pregnancy: Do's and Don'ts

As long as you're not considered high risk and you and your partner are comfortable, just about anything goes. But check out the sexual do's and don'ts below:

Oral Sex

Do: Have it. It's generally safe. If you're on the receiving end, take note (and mention it to him) that vaginal secretions may be heavier and may smell or taste different, though not necessarily unpleasantly so. If you're giving it, be warned that swallowing may increase nausea.

Don't: Allow him to blow air into your vagina. This can be very dangerous, causing a fatal air embolus.

Masturbation

Do: Know that it's safe during pregnancy. Because of increased blood flow in the genital region, your orgasms may be very intense or the area may be hypersensitive. You can use lubricants for added pleasure, and mutual masturbation can be a great substitute for intercourse.

Do: Use a vibrator if you'd like. It's safe, though the intense vibrations of an electrical vibrator may feel a little too intense and uncomfortable because of the increased blood flow to the vulva, clitoris, and vagina. You may find a battery-powered vibrator, with less intense vibrations, more to your liking.

Don't: Use vibrators inside the vagina after the second trimester.

continued

Anal Sex

Don't: It's probably best to avoid anal sex during pregnancy. The blood vessels surrounding the anus become dilated and more easily damaged during pregnancy. Some women have hemorrhoids, which may make anal sex uncomfortable. Plus, it's better not to risk spreading infection-causing bacteria from the rectum to the vagina.

Safe Sex

Do: Have it. It's even more important during pregnancy to protect you and the baby from sexually transmitted infections. If you have a new partner or if your partner is not monogamous, ask him to wear a condom.

is increasingly hard to find a comfortable position. During this time, you may ask your mate to simply hold you, massage you, or simply allow you to get a good night's sleep.

If you do muster up the energy and desire, sex may now be very awkward, since it'll prove difficult to find a comfortable position. But if you feel like having sex, try one of the positions mentioned previously or switch to oral sex or mutual masturbation.

As your body gets set for the delivery of your baby, you may feel more and more uncomfortable. Back pain, hemorrhoids, fatigue, breast leakage, varicose veins—all of these symptoms may lead to decreased desire. Intercourse, in particular, may lose its appeal. At this point, your vagina and vulva may feel "swollen." The baby's head drops during this trimester, creating pressure and discomfort during intercourse. If you have an orgasm—and it becomes more difficult to do this in this trimester—you may get contractions that last for several minutes and can be frightening, though not harmful. *However, you should call your doctor if your contractions last more than 30 minutes or are severe.* Some women may notice pink spotting after sex because of the increased swelling and softening of your cervix. *Though most likely not a problem, you should talk to your doctor immediately if you have spotting.*

Emotional Changes That May Affect Your Sexuality

As your due date nears, you and your mate may be very preoccupied with preparations for the baby, and you may feel like putting sex on the back burner. Also fear of harming the baby motivates many couples to give up sex completely. This is a natural response, though making love won't hurt your baby. At this point, however, you may need reassurance and cuddling from your partner rather than sex.

Postpartum Sexuality: After the Baby

Congratulations—you're a new mother. As soon as the bleeding has completely stopped and your vagina is not sore, you can resume sexual relations. But it's best to ask your doctor for advice. You'll need more time if you required an episiotomy, and even longer if you had a C-section and need to allow the abdominal incision to heal.

However, you may not feel very sexual. A new baby can be very demanding and time consuming, especially if this is your first. All new parents are tired, since babies require round-the-clock attention and care. Don't pressure yourself to return to an active sex life right away. Take your time and see how you and your mate are feeling as parents of a new baby. For some couples it takes more than a year to return to prepregnancy levels of sexual relations. You may want to express your love for your mate in other ways—and spend your few precious moments in bed actually sleeping—and reactivate your sexual lives once you feel more settled and less tired.

Physical Changes That May Affect Sexuality

Your body will feel quite different immediately after having a baby. Most women think that after the baby comes out, everything will be exactly the way it was before the little one was implanted inside. You may have had the experience of bringing some of your prepregnancy clothes to the hospital and being shocked when they didn't fit. It's shocking when you stand on the scale and find out that you've only lost 10 pounds—and the baby weighed 7 of those! Try to relax; your body will return to a state that is familiar to you.

Your breasts probably feel tender, and they've grown whether you've chosen to breast feed or not. You may want to ask him to avoid touching your breasts, at least at first, or to go gently.

Your vagina may feel different, and you may worry that labor and delivery have changed the size of your vagina so dramatically that you and your partner will no longer enjoy sexual intercourse. Don't worry, the vagina will return to normal size in time. Kegel exercises will help by building muscle tone, tightening the vagina, and increasing blood flow to the pelvic floor muscles. You can also try contracting your pelvic muscles during sex to increase stimulation. If you've had an episiotomy or trauma during delivery, your vagina may feel quite tender, and the thought of having intercourse may make you shiver with fear. Relax and take your time resuming sexual relations. Your vagina will heal and you will be able to enjoy intercourse again. In the meantime, if you are sore, find other delicious ways to enjoy each other sexually.

When you are ready to have sex for the first time since having the baby, make sure you slowly work up to intercourse. Spend lots of time on foreplay, stroking, massaging, and kissing each other to give your vagina time to lubricate and expand. Use lubricants the first few times to decrease the friction of the penis across your vaginal opening, and choose positions that take pressure off of your episiotomy and give you more control of where the penis goes: Woman-on-top positions are good when returning to intercourse after having a baby.

Don't be surprised if the sensations in your vagina are not as intense as they were prior to giving birth. It may take a few months for the nerves in your pelvis to recover. Orgasms, too, return slowly for most women, perhaps after several months.

Emotional Changes That May Affect Sexuality

After the baby, you might experience all sorts of new emotions. You may be worried about your ability to mother your baby, or you may be

Breast Feeding and Sex

Breast feeding is a healthy way to feed your baby and a wonderful way for you to bond with your newborn. Breast feeding, however, may affect your sex life.

The Prolactin Effect

Prolactin, the hormone that helps your body produce milk, may decrease your sex drive. That hormone can also depress sensation and make it more difficult to achieve orgasm.

Leaky Breasts

Expect your breasts to leak, especially during sex. This may be uncomfortable for you and your partner. Try feeding the baby before you have sex so that your breasts aren't as full. Or wear a bra with pads to bed.

Vaginal Dryness

During breast feeding, estrogen levels are low, which may cause vaginal dryness and painful intercourse. To combat this, try lubricants during intercourse or manual stimulation. In severe cases of dryness and atrophy (thinning), I sometimes recommend a tiny amount of estrogen cream.

continued

overwhelmed by all of your new responsibilities. You may also feel embarrassed about the changes in your body. Weak abdominal muscles, stretch marks, and stubborn pregnancy pounds can all wreak havoc with your self-esteem and desire. And having sex may make you feel guilty because deep down you feel that being a mother and making love can't go together. Relax, all of these feelings are normal. Your desire for sex will return to

Birth Control

It is possible to become pregnant while still breast feeding, so contraception is advised if you don't want to have another baby right away.

Sexual Feelings

Don't feel guilty if you have pleasurable sensations while breast feeding. Some women even have orgasms because of the intense nipple stimulation. Each of these experiences is normal and not at all sexual—kind of like a sneeze in response to your nose being tickled.

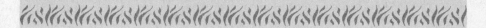

normal—though it may take up to one year. Remember that every woman's response is different, and you may find that you desire sex even more than before you became pregnant.

Postpartum depression is real and can put a damper on libido. If you're feeling particularly blue after the birth of your child, seek help from a professional.

Chapter 17
Of a Certain Age: Mature Sex

The day after my fortieth birthday I discovered that I needed reading glasses—the kind my grandmother wore. Other changes followed. My periods started coming closer together. I had difficulty remembering names. I developed acne, which I never had even as a teen! Every donut that I ate took the express train to my midsection. So began my *perimenopausal* years.

What Is Perimenopause?

Perimenopause is the time of transition that preceeds menopause. During this time your ovaries are producing less and less estrogen, and the levels may fluctuate wildly. Most women enter this phase of life in their mid-forties, though some women will begin as early as their late thirties. Perimenopause may last from two to ten years, and averages four years. You may have no detectable symptoms or complaints, or you may have a number of physical and psychological symptoms during this time.

Most, but not all, women reach their sexual peak in their mid-thirties and early forties. During this time, your libido may be at its highest level. You may crave sex more and find it more enjoyable than ever before. You may feel more secure in who you are, what your needs and desires are, and have fewer inhibitions about sex. If so, perimenopause can be a wonderful time for you. But not every woman has this experience. Some women may find that their desire for sex plummets at this time. Not only does their libido wane, they may even find sex uncomfortable. Still other women have no noticeable change in their sexual desire.

Let's look at some of the changes and common complaints that affect a woman's sex life during the important perimenopause transition period.

My vagina is dry.

Changes in your vaginal secretions can start years before menopause. You may notice that it takes much longer for you to become wet, and you may not produce as much lubrication as you did in the past. As a result, sexual intercourse may become more uncomfortable. Sometimes you may appear to be wet enough but find that the lubrication does not last long enough so that you become dry and sore before intercourse ends. Your partner may also notice the change in your secretions and mistakenly assume that you are not as interested in sex. He may feel rejected and withdraw from sexual activity. You may also fear that something is wrong with you and/or your relationship.

What to Do

Accept that changes in your secretions are normal and do not signal that something is wrong. Discuss your natural physical changes with your partner and work together as a team to make sure your sex life remains satisfying. Use water-based lubricants for masturbation or intercourse. For intercourse, lubricants work best if you spread it on his penis as well as inside your vagina.

Is it hot in here, or is it me?

Hot flashes may start years before your very last menstrual period, although some women never experience them. For those who do, hot flashes can be distressing.

As you age, your ovaries begin to make less and less estrogen. Though nobody knows for sure what causes hot flashes, physicians think that the decrease in estrogen levels causes your internal "thermostat" to go haywire, causing your blood vessels to dilate and your face and upper body to flush. Most women experience hot flashes as waves of heat that radiate from the chest, neck, face, and head. You may also have sweating with your flashes; and when it occurs at night they are called *night sweats*. Night sweats can soak your sheets and interfere with your sleep. Hot flashes, night sweats, and fatigue caused by sleep problems can throw a ringer in your desire and enjoyment of sex. You may find that you just don't have enough energy for lovemaking.

What to Do

Birth control pills provide the estrogen that you are lacking and will relieve hot flashes. Estrogen replacement therapy may be started when it is clear that menopause is imminent. Talk to your doctor about the risks and benefits of estrogen therapy. Natural supplements such as black cohosh (Remifemin), soy supplements, evening primrose oil, red clover (Promensil), and chasteberry may also provide relief and are natural alternatives to hormones. A healthy diet that avoids foods that trigger hot flashes, such as alcohol, coffee, and colas; vitamins; and regular exercise can help to alleviate hot flashes. And because you may have the need to shed some clothes quickly during a flash, dress in layers.

Middle-age Spread

As you age, your metabolism begins to slow. That means that, to maintain the same weight, you will need to either decrease the number of calories you consume every day or increase the number of calories you burn by increasing your activities. To add insult to injury, when you put on weight, it settles in your abdomen. You may develop a slight bulge in your midsection even if you exercise and cut calories.

The Need for Contraception

Some women assume that because their periods are changing they are no longer fertile and can't conceive. While it is true that you may not ovulate every month during this transition, and your fertility is lower than it was when you were twenty, you may become pregnant during the months that you do ovulate. If you do not want to have a baby at this time, you will need to use contraceptives until you have not had a period for one year, or your blood tests consistently suggest that you are no longer ovulating.

For most women, weight increases as you approach menopause. In fact it is the number-one complaint of middle-aged women in my practice. As your body changes, you may start to fear that you no longer appear sexy, attractive, and desirable. Your self-esteem can plummet, and if you feel uncomfortable with your body, it will be difficult to enjoy sex.

What to Do

Eat a low-fat healthy diet and increase your activities. Begin an exercise program that includes weight training and aerobics. Improving your strength and stamina and toning your body will make you feel more confident and improve your libido. It also helps to accept the fact that you will never have the body of a sixteen-year-old again, so learn to appreciate and love the wonderful body that you have.

Who moved my libido?

Diminished desire for sex is one of the most common complaints I hear from women nearing menopause. As your ovaries age, they produce less testosterone—the hormone of desire—which is responsible for your libido as well as sexual enjoyment. Of course other concerns that sometimes increase as we approach menopause, such as vaginal dryness, stress, anxiety, mood swings, and relationship issues, can also affect your desire for sex.

What to Do

Treating your vaginal dryness alone may make sex more comfortable and increase your desire. Ask your doctor to test your testosterone level, and if your testosterone is low, testosterone supplements may boost your desire and enjoyment of sex.

Menopause (The Change)

Menopause is not a disease. It is a natural part of every woman's life that signals the end of your childbearing years. Like puberty, it is filled with changes in your body, emotions, and hormones. Despite the horror stories and myths that pervade our culture, menopause should be celebrated as the end of one phase of our lives and the beginning of a potentially more fulfilling one. And as long as you are healthy, sex can be a significant and special part of your life—if you want it to be. Don't let anyone pressure you into being sexual if that is not what you want. On the other hand, don't let anyone tell you that you are past the age for sexual activity.

With menopause, your ovaries stop releasing eggs and you stop having menstrual periods. You are considered postmenopausal when you have not had a natural period for one year. The average age of menopause in the United States is fifty-two, but 1 percent of women experience premature menopause before the age of forty. You also become menopausal when your ovaries are surgically removed, most commonly at the time of hysterectomy.

Menopause may bring new and different symptoms and changes in your body. It is important to keep in mind that all women are different and that some will have no annoying symptoms during or after menopause. In fact some women find this time of life to be the most enjoyable. You may find that you are more self-assured and confident. You know who you are, what you want, and how to get it. You may feel empowered, knowledgeable, strong, and creative.

Sex during menopause can be better than ever. And some women have a marked increase in their sex drive during this time. With age and experience, you may be less concerned about sexual taboos and know what turns you on. Menopause removes the fear of pregnancy—no more condoms, pills, or diaphragms—which can be very liberating. Sex can be more spontaneous and relaxed. If the children have left the nest, you have more privacy: You can have sex in the kitchen, living room, or in the backyard. Other women, however, may experience no change or a dip in sexual desire during menopause—and that too is normal.

Physical Changes

With the loss of estrogen, your genitals undergo changes, the extent of which will vary from one woman to the next. In some women the changes are so minor as to be barely noticeable; other women may experience more dramatic changes. Let's look at some of the possibilities.

Your Vulva

Your mons and labia may become thinner and lose their fullness, and your pubic hair may become sparse and gray. If your clitoris is more exposed with these changes, it may become very sensitive to touch.

Your Clitoris

As blood flow decreases, your clitoris becomes smaller, and it may take longer for your clitoris to become engorged during arousal. You may have less sensitivity, and some menopausal women have described the clitoris as "dead." These changes in your clitoris may make it more difficult for you to climax—requiring more time—and your orgasms may not be as intense as they were before menopause.

Your Vagina

The blood flow to your vagina decreases, too. As a result, it may take longer for your vagina to become wet when you are aroused, and you may produce less moisture than you did prior to menopause. Your vagina may feel dry, itchy, and irritated. The walls of the vagina become thin, smooth, and less elastic, and sometimes the vaginal walls "weep," producing a thin, watery discharge.

Without estrogen, the pH of the vagina changes—from an acidic environment to a more alkaline one—as do the natural bacteria that live there. Consequently, you may become more prone to infection. The loss of acidity in your vagina may cause burning when your partner ejaculates because you are unable to neutralize his alkaline semen. Last, the odor of your vagina may change. It won't become offensive, just different.

Your Uterus

There is a decrease in the blood flow to your uterus and it, too, becomes smaller.

Your Breasts

Your breasts may become larger and softer. The glands in your breasts are replaced with fat, and your breasts may lose their firmness. You may find that your nipples have lost some of their sensitivity and are less responsive during sex.

Your Bladder

The tissue lining your bladder and urethra thin. You may begin to lose urine when you cough, sneeze, or during sex. Changes in the lining of your bladder make infections more common, especially after sex.

Making Sex Better After Menopause

You can make your vagina plush and moist with estrogen replacement therapy. Estrogen increases the blood flow to your vagina, vulva, clitoris, bladder, and urethra, decreasing the pain that comes with vaginal dryness and increasing the sensitivity of your clitoris. Should you decide to take estrogen, your doctor will prescribe a combination of an estrogen and a progesterone hormone (unless you no longer have a uterus, in which case you don't need progesterone). Both hormones can be taken in the form of a pill or a patch. If loss of libido is also a problem, your doctor may prescribe Estratest, a combination of estrogen and testosterone, in addition to progesterone. Discuss all options with your doctor.

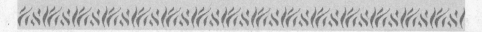

More Reasons to Stop Smoking

Smoking accelerates the onset of menopause and increases hot flashes and night sweats. It also decreases blood flow to your vagina, making it drier and sex more uncomfortable. Cigarette smoking can depress your libido, arousal, and orgasms. And I'm sure you are aware that it increases your risks of genital cancers among others.

Occasionally, even with estrogen replacement therapy, the vagina will remain dry enough to make sex uncomfortable. Adding an estrogen cream (applied with an applicator inside your vagina) to your hormone replacement therapy, or using the cream alone, can help to make your vagina moist. You may notice improvement after only a few weeks of therapy, though sometimes several months are needed to reverse the changes of menopause. Estrogen also comes in a tablet form (Vagifem) that is placed in your vagina two to three times a week, and in a vaginal ring that remains in your vagina for three months (Estring). I sometimes recommend massaging a small pea-sized amount of estrogen cream directly into the tissue of the vagina and vulva. Massaging it into the tissues means that you will need to use less estrogen, and the act of massaging helps to increase blood flow and strengthen the tissue. Vitamin E oil or oil of St. John's wort may be used for massage instead of estrogen if you desire. Massage is also wonderful because touching your genitals puts you in touch with your body and the many pleasurable sensations that it holds.

If you can't or do not want to use estrogen, a vaginal moisturizer such as Replens can be used three times a week to keep the vagina moist, or you can spread a small amount of Crisco (the kind in the tub, not the oil) on your labia daily to keep them moist and to relieve the itching and irritation you sometimes get from a dry vulva.

Try a variety of water-based lubricants for intercourse and masturbation. Lubricants make intercourse more pleasurable and can be a lot of fun! Make a game of stroking, touching, and massaging each other with the lubricants as a buildup to intercourse. Two slippery surfaces are better than one.

Menopause is a good time to experiment more with new sexual positions. Positions that give you more control of the depth of penetration and tempo of sex will make it more comfortable for you.

Spend more time building up to intercourse by hugging, kissing, massaging, and orally stimulating your vagina to give it the extra time it needs to get moist after menopause. Or skip intercourse altogether and spend time discovering new erogenous zones and ways of obtaining mutual sexual pleasure. There is no one right way to be sexual. The intimacy of touch and physical closeness can be as satisfying, if not more so, as intercourse. In fact, for many women it is preferable.

Experiment with different methods of touching your clitoris. Do you like soft, hard, direct, or indirect touch? Show your partner what feels good to you. If you don't already own a vibrator, buy one. The increased stimulation of the vibrator provides the intense stimulation that you sometimes need after menopause.

You can prevent some of the changes in your vagina by remaining sexually active after menopause. Vaginal intercourse, masturbation, fantasy, erotic massage, or any other activity that arouses you and gives you sexual pleasure can help to keep your vagina moist, soft, and healthy. If intercourse is important to you now or will be in the future, having regular intercourse (once a week or more) or placing a dildo, vibrator, dilator, or two to three fingers in your vagina while masturbating once a week will prevent the shortening and shrinking of your vagina that can occur over time when estrogen is lacking. Kegel exercises have also been shown to be effective in keeping your vagina toned and elastic.

Discuss the changes in your sexual desire and response with your partner. You may need to make some changes in how you relate to each other sexually, but that doesn't mean that your sex life together need be any less satisfying for the two of you. There is a world of satisfying sexual possibilities to explore.

Interesting Fact

Studies show that when menopausal women begin a relationship with a new, interesting, and interested partner, sexual problems disappear. Sexual desire, frequency, and enjoyment skyrocket (especially if the partner is younger). No, I'm not recommending that you trade your old one in for a new model, but if you are single and afraid to enter a new relationship because you think you are "all dried up," you should give it a whirl.

The Male Menopause: Midlife Crisis

Not only women undergo significant changes during the midlife years. Gail Sheehy, author of *Understanding Men's Passages: Discovering the New Map of Men's Lives*, describes the midlife changes in men as MANopause. Common symptoms of MANopause include irritability, decreased energy, and mood swings. According to Ms. Sheehy, testosterone levels decrease by 1 percent per year after age forty. The penis begins to become sluggish, and many men in their forties begin to notice some difficulty attaining and maintaining their erections. After the age of fifty, it is not uncommon for men occasionally to have partial erections or difficulty reaching orgasm.

Changes in sexual performance may cause anxiety, shame, and depression. Sex becomes less desired and less frequent, and sometimes men will withdraw from intimacy altogether. Most women will become distressed and assume that her partner's lack of interest in sex is a signal that he no longer finds her desirable. She begins to feel insecure and rejected. She may even fear that he has found someone else.

Men may also have sexual difficulty because of their fear of hurting you. And if menopausal changes have made your vagina difficult to enter with a less-than-optimal erection, he may lose his desire for sexual intercourse.

Again, communication with your partner is important. Share your concerns and don't be afraid to seek professional counseling if needed.

Libido Issues

Our culture places a great emphasis on youth. For some of us, it is difficult to accept the natural physical changes that come with age. We begin to fear that we are no longer attractive, sexy, or desirable. We may no longer feel comfortable allowing others to see and touch certain parts of our body. Loss of self-esteem kills libido.

Your relationship with your partner can also be responsible for changes in your libido, as can the stresses of children, aging parents, work, career, homemaking, illness, and medications. You may find that after taking care of everybody else, there is little energy left for even the thought of sex.

Viagra: Friend or Foe?

Viagra can be a wonder drug when male erectile dysfunction makes mutually desired intercourse impossible. One tiny pill can provide him with a strong youthful erection. But it is sometimes forgotten that the vagina of a woman changes after years of disuse and lack of estrogen. If it has been a number of years since you last had intercourse, you may need to prepare your vagina before sex. Several weeks of estrogen therapy and/or massages using vitamin E oil will help to soften, stretch, and strengthen your vagina. In some cases, well-lubricated dilators or dildos may be required to slowly stretch the delicate tissues. Be patient. It's never too late to begin an active sex life.

Chapter 18

More Than Birds and Bees: Talking to Your Daughter About Sex

Amy was fifteen years old and scared. The itching and burning near her vagina had become unbearable, so she finally told her mother and they came to see me. Her mother told me that her daughter had a "yeast infection" but asked me not to use a speculum to examine Amy because she was a virgin.

When I examined Amy, I found growths covering the opening to her vagina and her labia. She also had a large open sore on her vulva. Her hymenal ring was small and intact, so she was, in fact, technically a virgin—but she was infected with herpes and covered with warts, two sexually transmitted diseases. When I informed her, she told me that she had not had sex but had allowed her boyfriend to rub against her with his pants down. "He never went inside me," she cried. "Please don't tell my mom!"

The teen world is full of myths and misinformation about sex. In my practice I have seen many young women with serious sexually transmitted diseases and a few technical virgins who were actually pregnant.

Why Do You Need to Talk to Your Daughter About Sex?

Amy is a composite of several teens I have seen over the years. These cases and others are excellent examples of why we must talk to our daughters about sex. Not only about the anatomy and the way things work but also about self-esteem and the right to say "no" to unwanted sexual contact. Each of these girls had intimate contact to please their boyfriends. None of them felt ready to have intercourse but made the compromise of having outercourse or oral or anal sex. None of them felt confident enough to say "no." And it is self-confidence that enables a teenage girl to choose healthy and self-nurturing behaviors.

Talking to your daughter will give her the knowledge she needs and empower her to make good decisions. Through communication, we can break the cycle of misinformation, sexual myths, low sexual self-esteem, and sexual dysfunction for our daughters. We can help them have a good start toward a healthy and satisfying sex life as adults. It is our responsibility.

Preparing to Talk About Sex

Talking about sex is not always easy. In fact, for many, it can be embarrassing and uncomfortable. If you and your mother never talked about sex, or if most of the messages you received about sex were negative, it can be especially difficult to broach the subject with your daughter. You may not know how to initiate the conversation and fear that you will not do it right. The following tips might help you prepare.

🌿 There are many good books available to give you guidance, and my favorites are listed in the resources section of this book. Choose books that are deemed appropriate for your daughter's age and circumstances. Read the books alone, and if you find them appropriate and consistent with your values, set aside private time to read them to, or with, your daughter. Encourage your daughter to ask questions and avoid using this as an opportunity to lecture.

🌿 Ask your child's pediatrician for advice. They can tell you what issues they are confronting in your daughter's age group and share some ideas about how to broach them.

🌿 Organize your thoughts. Sometimes it helps to prepare for talking to your daughter by deciding ahead of time the messages that you want to get across to her. Write them down and practice what you will say if you feel that would make it easier for you to bring up an uncomfortable topic.

Facing Your Fears

Fear That You Won't Know the Answers

There is no need to be embarrassed if you don't feel that you have the knowledge to teach your daughter all that she needs to know about sex. Most women don't get a formal sex education, and few of us received detailed sex information from our mothers. You don't have to be an expert to help your children get answers to their questions. It is enough to let them know that you will always be there to help them look for those answers.

Fear That Talking About Sex Will Lead to Sex

It is a common misconception that talking about sex will encourage girls to become sexually active at an early age. You may fear that open and honest discussions about sex may be interpreted by your daughter as giving permission to indulge. Multiple studies have shown that girls who receive sex information from their mothers are more likely to delay intercourse than those left to their own devices. When they do become sexually active, girls armed with accurate information are more likely to use contraceptives, protect themselves against sexually transmitted diseases, and avoid risky sex behavior. Knowledge is power, and information helps girls make good decisions. Besides, if you don't discuss sex with your daughter, someone else will. And the messages that person gives may be incorrect, confusing, and inconsistent with your family values.

Sometimes we mistakenly assume that if we don't talk about it, it won't happen. If only life were that simple. Keeping silent may give her the message that she can't talk to you about sex or any other intimate personal issues.

Fear of Making a Mistake

No matter how well informed you might be, it is still possible to make mistakes. No one is perfect. Just do the best you can. Let me share another story with you. When my daughter was two years old I noticed her happily exploring her vulva. I asked her why she was touching herself. "Because it feels good," she said. (If only we could maintain that innocence.) I wish I could say that I handled this situation in the right way. I wish I could say that I told her that it was okay to touch herself. But something deep inside me felt uncomfortable, and without thinking, I grabbed her hand away. She gave me a puzzled look and started to cry. I then realized what I had done and I apologized. I apologized again ten years later during one of our girl talks about sex and sexuality. "It's okay, Mom," she said, and we hugged.

Negotiating Those Early Years

Teaching your daughter about sex is an ongoing process. It begins at birth and continues years past adolescence. The messages you give in the early years may follow her into adulthood and affect how she feels about her body and her sexuality. The following points may help you in your early instruction.

Give Your Daughter Correct Names
for Her Sexual Anatomy

Most of us tell our daughters the names of all of their body parts but neglect to tell them the correct names for their sexual anatomy. Debra Haffner, author of *From Diapers to Dating*, suggests that you may be inadvertently giving your daughter the message that this part of her body (her sexual anatomy) has no name, is different from the rest of her body, and should not be discussed.

Using terms like "down there," "privates," "coochie," or "stink hole" make a girl feel even more disconnected from and even ashamed of her body. These feelings can sometimes affect her feelings in adulthood and make it more difficult for her to enjoy sex. Early on, tell her about her vulva and vagina. As she gets older, you will want to introduce labia and clitoris. When she is ready, you might want to show her how to use a mirror to look at the hidden parts of her sexual anatomy and begin to talk about how her genitals function. If it is uncomfortable for you or your daughter to perform this exercise, don't force it. She may decide to take a look at another time in private—and that is okay.

The average age for the first menstrual period is between eleven and twelve years. Begin to talk about the changes that she can expect in her body long before she starts her menses, as early as eight years according to experts. Remember to be positive in presenting information about this special time in a girl's life.

Exploring Her Genitals Is Normal

You may have noticed that babies, girls and boys, love to touch themselves from the time they are infants. You take off the diaper and the hands go straight between their legs. Children like to explore and learn about all of the parts of their bodies, and touching the genitals feels good.

It is very common for mothers to feel uncomfortable when their daughters touch themselves. Moms often worry that this innocent investigation represents sexual interest or will lead to early sexual experimentation. Self-exploration by small children is not at all sexual. Taking your daughter's hands away or raising your voice to tell her to stop may give her the message that her genitals are dirty or bad. Such messages may inadvertently cause her to have feelings of shame, guilt, and discomfort with her body that last a lifetime.

And as your daughter gets older, keep in mind that masturbation is normal and causes no harm. If she is stimulating herself in public, however, let her know that masturbation is normal but should be done in private.

Protect Her from Abuse

Experts suggest that you start talking to your daughter about sex abuse when she reaches the age of preschool. Tell her that her body is private and special and, most important, that it is her own. A girl should be taught that no one has the right to touch her—especially in the genital area—or ask her to do anything that makes her feel uncomfortable.

Strategies for Talking to Your Older Children About Sex

Give Accurate Information

When your child asks questions, give honest and accurate information. The answers should be brief, accurate, and tailored to your child's age. Answering questions about sex honestly, openly, and in a warm, matter-of-fact manner will give the message that sexuality is normal and natural.

Be an "Askable Parent"

Let your daughter know that you are always available and enthusiastic about answering her questions. If possible, try to answer the question at the time that your child asks. Do not tell her that you'll answer it when she is older. If you don't know the answer to her question, don't fudge it or ignore it. Admit that you don't know the answer and promise to look it up and get back to her with the answer. You might also consider using this as an opportunity for the two of you to increase your mother-daughter bond by researching the answer together.

Be a Good Listener

As difficult as it may be to talk to your daughter about sex, it may be even more difficult to listen. I mean *really* listen. It's sometimes easier to lecture our daughters than to listen to their points of view. It is important to let your daughter discuss her feelings and attitudes about everything, including sex.

Be Aware of "Teachable Moments"

Listen for opportunities to teach your daughter about sex. Some girls will ask a lot of questions, but others will ask none. If you wait for her to ask before you start talking about sex, you may never get the chance to give her the knowledge that she needs to grow up confident and secure with her body and sexuality. Learn to take advantage of what child development experts call "teachable moments." You may not realize it, but teachable moments are all around you. Television programs, articles in the newspapers, and songs on the radio may all provide lead-ins to a discussion about sex.

Share Your Values

Girls need, and want, to know your values. It is important that you share your feelings, beliefs, and attitudes regarding sex. It is equally important that you tell your daughter why you feel the way that you do. Telling her she must do something "because I say so" is not going to give her the knowledge and self-esteem that she will need when she must make her own decisions. Your values will help your daughter establish her own boundaries, and boundaries are what keep her safe.

Be Sex Positive

I don't mean that you should be a "cheerleader" for sex, or that you should encourage your daughter to go out and experiment. I do mean that you need to give her positive messages about sex that fit in with your values. Let her know that sex can be beautiful in a loving committed relationship (or in marriage, if that is what you believe). Girls who receive sex-positive messages while growing up are more likely to become women who are comfortable and confident in their sexuality as adults. If you only tell her about the dangers of sex and none of the joys, she may never have a positive adult sexual experience.

Celebrating Menstruation

One of the most important milestones of a girl's teen and preteen years is the start of her menstrual period. Do you remember the day you first had yours? Was it a positive experience? For many of us, the start of our menstrual periods was met with apprehension, embarrassment, and fear. The words we use to describe the menses—"the curse," "the plague," "on the rag," for instance—make a girl feel bad about what should be a positive experience. She may develop feelings of shame and embarrassment, and she may begin to feel bad about her body, femininity, and sexuality.

For centuries the beginning of menstruation has been celebrated in other cultures. Girls are welcomed into the "circle of womanhood" with traditional ceremonies. You can give your daughter the same positive message by planning something special to celebrate her first menstruation. You can buy her a special gift; have a celebratory dinner, tea, or lunch together; or take a mother-daughter trip.

Building Strong Mother-Daughter Bonds

Girls who have strong bonds and good communication with their mothers are more likely to be sexually healthy. So as your daughter grows up, make sure to spend some "girl time" with her. Girl time can consist of a few minutes at bedtime every day or a special hour on the weekend. Use the time to talk and listen.

Read your daughter stories and books about female leaders and heroes. Share positive, uplifting stories about yourself and other women in your family. Daughters love to hear stories about how their mothers handled the perils of childhood and adolescence. This kind of intimate sharing can help her develop a sense of self-worth and pride. And through your private conversations she will learn communication and decision-making skills. Have fun, laugh together, and don't forget to hug.

More Than the Birds and the Bees

As important as it is to discuss pregnancy prevention and protection against sexually transmitted infections, it is equally important to discuss the emotional side of sex. Be sure to speak honestly with your daughter about sex, love, and the importance of developing committed, positive, honest, and loving relationships. Also, be certain to reassure her. Teens will experience strong sexual feelings and thoughts. Let her know that what she is feeling is normal but that she doesn't have to act on it. Discuss the many ways that you can show love and affection without having sex. Give her permission and the courage to say "no," and the wisdom to know when to say "yes."

Discussions about sexual behavior and orientation are also important. Few mothers discuss oral sex, anal sex, masturbation, and homosexuality with their daughters. But if you don't think these conversations are important, think again. A *New York Times* article in 2000 revealed that oral sex is considered an acceptable and safe activity, like a good-night kiss, for some children in middle school.

Talking and listening to your daughter and keeping the lines of communication open throughout her life will help her to grow up to be a sexually healthy and confident woman. Not only will she have a good chance of experiencing the intimacy, pleasure, and satisfaction that healthy sexuality can provide, but the two of you will build a wonderfully trusting relationship.

Part V

When Sex Isn't Great

Chapter 19

Medical Problems

In my medical practice, I've met many women who don't fit into the neat categories of "dysfunction," but who are unhappy with their sex lives at least part of the time. A full 43 percent of women have some form of sexual dysfunction, according to the National Health and Social Life Survey, a study of adult sexual behavior in the United States. Women may be dissatisfied with sex for several reasons. To better understand what can go wrong, let's look at the traditional model of the female sexual response cycle (initially described by Masters and Johnson and later modified by Dr. Helen Kaplan).

The Female Sexual Response Cycle

Desire

Desire is the feeling of motivation to seek out or be willing to participate in sex.

Arousal

Though arousal is often considered the second stage of sexual response, it is possible for women to experience arousal before desire, and sometimes the two occur simultaneously. The first sign of arousal is lubrication of your vagina, which may begin to happen within seconds of physical or psychological stimulation, though you may not yet feel excited. As you become more sexually excited, blood flow increases to your genitals, increasing the size of your clitoris and labia. Your cervix and uterus move up in your pelvis, causing your vagina to become longer and wider at the top. As the lower part of your vagina swells, it decreases in size and forms what is called the "orgasmic platform," the part that will contract when you have an orgasm. Your nipples become erect, and your breasts increase in size. At the height of excitement, your clitoris retracts under the hood to prevent overstimulation, sometimes seeming to disappear.

Orgasm

Orgasm is a total-body experience. Your heart rate, blood pressure, and rate of breathing increase, and if stimulation is intense enough and lasts long enough, you may experience intensely pleasurable contractions of your uterus, orgasmic platform, pelvic floor muscles, and anal sphincter. The contractions occur at 0.8-second intervals, and most women experience between 3 and 15 contractions. If stimulation and interest continue after the first orgasm, it is possible for some women to have an unlimited number of additional orgasms.

Resolution

The swelling and engorgement eases, and your breasts, labia, vagina, and clitoris return to their usual size. Resolution may take seconds or up to 1 hour.

Why is the sexual response cycle important? According to the experts, problems with any stage of the sexual response cycle can cause what is called *sexual dysfunction*—the inability to enjoy sex. Sexual dysfunction is divided into four major categories: *hypoactive sexual desire disorder, sexual arousal disorder, orgasmic disorder,* and *sexual pain disorder.*

Female Sexual Dysfunction: Definitions

Hypoactive Sexual Desire Disorder

If you consistently lack sexual thoughts and fantasies, have no desire or motivation for sex, or are not open or responsive to the advances of your lover, you may have desire disorder. In order to be classified as such, you also must experience personal distress about your situation. For example, if you find your lack of desire acceptable, even if your partner doesn't, it is not considered sexual dysfunction but a relationship issue. According to the National Health and Social Life Survey, one-third of women lack the desire for sex. Similarly, if you are phobic about sex and totally avoid it with a partner—and it causes personal distress—you have a related dysfunction: *sexual aversion disorder.*

Sexual Arousal Disorder

If you consistently have problems getting aroused or excited about sex or if you have problems with vaginal lubrication and engorgement of your genitals and either is causing you personal distress, you have sexual arousal disorder.

Orgasmic Disorder

If you have recurrent difficulty achieving orgasm despite being aroused and sufficiently stimulated, and it causes you personal distress, you have orgasmic disorder.

Sexual Pain Disorder

This category of dysfunction may manifest itself in a variety of ways: *Dyspareunia* is recurrent genital pain with intercourse. *Vaginismus* is recurrent spasms of the outer vagina that interfere with your ability to have intercourse and cause pain and personal distress. *Noncoital sexual pain disorder* is recurrent genital pain during sexual activities other than intercourse.

. . .

A woman may not be satisfied with her sex life because of one or more of the above sexual disorders. As a gynecologist, however, I don't like to say that a woman who is not enjoying her sex life is "dysfunctional," "abnormal," or "disordered." True, women may have problems with sexual enjoyment for medical or psychological reasons, or both, but sometimes sexual dissatisfaction has nothing at all to do with a "dysfunction." Sonia, for instance, never has fantasies or spontaneous desire for sex. "I never feel horny," she says. However, she can become aroused if the right opportunity for sex presents itself. She was satisfied with her sex life until she read an article that suggested that she was abnormal, and now she is distressed. Lisa, on the other hand, becomes aroused and has orgasms—so there's nothing wrong with her physically—but because of problems in her relationship, she doesn't find sex with her partner satisfying.

The bottom line: Sexual dissatisfaction may be caused by medical problems, medications, surgery, psychological or cultural issues, partner or relationship problems as well as the changes that normally occur during the various stages of life.

Illnesses That Can Put a Damper on Your Sex Life

When you are not feeling well, sex moves lower on your list of priorities. Pain, weakness, fatigue, and depression are libido busters and may make it difficult for you to enjoy sex. Chronic medical problems also can affect your sense of yourself as a sexual being; they can affect the entire female sexual response cycle as well.

Having a chronic medical problem does not mean that you must give up your sex life. You may need to make adjustments to your usual approach to sex, but rest assured, the pleasure can be as satisfying as before.

In the following pages, I cover the problems I often help my patients to confront. If any of these issues are yours, be sure to pay special attention to my advice on what to do to fully reclaim your sexual self.

What to Do If You Have a Chronic Medical Problem

Consult Your Doctor

Don't be embarrassed to raise sexual issues with your doctor. She or he can give you the guidance you need to continue an active sex life and perhaps make it better. Be sure to find out exactly when you can resume sexual activity, which activities are safe, and what your limitations are. If your doctor can't talk frankly about sex, ask for an informed and knowledgeable referral. Include your partner, if you have one, in the discussions.

Improve Your General Health

Exercise and a healthy diet are essential for satisfying sex. Avoid smoking and excessive alcohol consumption.

Remember That Sex Is More Than Intercourse

Some medical problems may interfere, temporarily or permanently, with your ability to have intercourse. There are many ways to express yourself sexually and continue a satisfying sex life. Experiment and use your imagination.

Choose the Right Location for Sex

A room that is too hot, cold, or humid can be stressful to your body.

Choose the Best Times for Sex

Sex is best when you are well rested. Choose the time of day when you have the most energy, even if it means having sex in the middle of the day.

continued

Likewise, the time when you are most likely to be pain free would be best for intimacy.

Get in a Good Position for Love

Choose positions that do not strain your muscles and joints or place pressure on sensitive body parts.

Take Care of Your Vagina

Many medical problems will interfere with the ability of your vagina to lubricate and will cause dryness. Use a water-based lubricant and spend lots of time on foreplay to improve vaginal moisture.

Heart Disease and Sex

The most common way people react when they have been diagnosed with heart disease, especially after a heart attack, is to stop having sex regularly, if at all. The normal signs of sexual arousal—increased heart rate, sweating, and rapid breathing—may now be misinterpreted as signs of an impending heart problem. Fear that sex may cause chest pain, heart attack, or death can destroy your libido. Your partner also may be fearful of intimacy and the effect that making love may have on your heart. In some men, these fears may lead to impotence. Suddenly a healthy, active sex life may become infrequent and anxiety provoking. No wonder most women who've had a heart attack experience a loss of desire for sex and problems with arousal and orgasm.

Having heart disease doesn't have to ruin your sex life. The risk of having a heart attack during or after sex is actually very low—about 20 chances per million in patients with heart disease, about the same as the risk of having a heart attack after a fit of anger.

What to Do

Consult Your Doctor: With your doctor's guidance, it is possible to continue to have an active and satisfying sex life. *If you've had a heart attack or heart surgery, make sure you get clearance from your doctor before engaging in any sexual activity; sex before your heart heals can be dangerous.* Remember, doctors are human—and most of them have sex as well—so don't be shy about broaching the subject. If your doctor can't talk frankly about sex, ask for an informed and knowledgeable referral. Be sure to include your partner (if you have one) in all discussions about sex.

Most doctors equate the energy required for an average 15-minute sexual encounter with the energy you'd need to climb two flights of stairs at the rate of two stairs per second. If you have no chest pain or prolonged breathlessness after you reach the top, you can safely have sex.

Your doctor might recommend a treadmill stress test to check your sexual fitness. Your doctor will monitor your heart as you walk briskly on a treadmill to be sure you can handle the physical exertion of sex. Another helpful test for alleviating your anxieties about resuming your sex life is the "sexercise tolerance test." For this, you will be required to wear a Holter monitor for 24 hours. The monitor will let your doctor know exactly how your heart responds during all your daily activities, including sex.

Your doctor may prescribe medications that lower the risks of injuring your heart during sex. Discuss timing your medications so they are most effective during the times you are most likely to have sex.

Exercise Regularly: Ask your doctor to prescribe a program that is safe for you. Exercise strengthens your heart so it works more efficiently during sex. When you are physically fit, your heart doesn't need to beat as rapidly during sex, and you're less likely to experience pain or discomfort.

Time Your Sexual Encounters: Wait at least three hours after a heavy meal or alcohol before having sex. Digestion of a heavy meal places extra demands on your heart.

Get in a Good Position for Love: Studies show that woman-on-top, man-on-top, and side-to-side positions are safe. If you are on top, allow your partner to assume most of your body weight.

Know What's Safe: Once your doctor gives you the go-ahead to resume your sex life, you can participate in oral sex, masturbation, or intercourse. The jury is still out about anal sex. Some doctors worry that stretching the nerves in and around the anus can cause a slowing of your heart. Spend lots of time on foreplay so your heart rate increases gradually.

Report to Your Doctor: If sexual activity causes chest pain, rapid heart rate, or shortness of breath lasting more than several minutes after orgasm, or if it causes extreme fatigue, call your doctor.

Hypertension (High Blood Pressure) and Sex

Though most women have no sexual side effects from the disease, hypertension can interfere with your ability to enjoy sex. It can damage your blood vessels and decrease the flow of blood throughout your body, including your vagina. It may become more difficult for your vagina to become wet during sex, causing pain during intercourse. Your ability to orgasm may likewise be affected. Some medications used to treat high blood pressure also can cause problems with your sexual desire and performance.

What to Do

If your blood pressure is very high and not controlled by medications or other means, consult your doctor about the safety of sex. If the medications are causing sexual side effects, speak frankly with your doctor so that a substitute medication can be found.

Diabetes and Sex

Most women with diabetes will notice no change in their sexuality. For other women, vaginal dryness, chronic vaginal infections, and urinary-tract infections can cause pain and discomfort during sex. If sex is uncomfortable, it's unlikely you'll desire it. The incidence of sexual problems sometimes increases the longer you have diabetes, because the disease may affect your nerves and blood vessels, weakening the sensations in your vagina and clitoris.

What to Do

Some people have a carbohydrate snack before sex to avoid a drop in sugar levels during sex, but sex causes only a mild, insignificant drop in your glucose level. So, if your diabetes is well under control, there is no need for the snack precaution. Chronic vaginal infections with yeast are very common in women with diabetes. If you have a yeast infection, sex can be painful and may exacerbate the infection. Antifungal creams should be applied to your vulva and vagina. To stem repeat yeast infections, try natural treatments such as acidophilus, garlic tablets, and yogurt. Urinate both before and soon after sex to decrease your chances of a bladder infection.

If you have developed neuropathy (nerve damage) as a complication of your diabetes, you may need more stimulation of your clitoris and vagina for satisfying sex. Adding a vibrator to masturbation and to sex with a partner may give you the added zip you need.

Epilepsy and Sex

Seizure disorders have been shown to cause problems with sexual arousal and vaginal lubrication, and many seizure medications have been shown to cause sexual dysfunction (though most studies have only been done on men).

What to Do

Talk to your doctor about your medication. In some cases, changing your dose or type of medication will improve your libido and arousal.

Multiple Sclerosis and Sex

With multiple sclerosis, you sometimes may feel lusty and sexual and at other times you may have problems with arousal, difficulty achieving orgasm, or just no desire for sex at all. Muscle weakness and spasms can make sexual intercourse difficult, and changes in the sensations in your genitals can interfere with your sexual pleasure. If you have problems controlling your bowels or urine, you may avoid sex for fear of an embarrassing loss of control.

What to Do

Medications used to treat the symptoms of multiple sclerosis may interfere with sexual enjoyment. Talk to your doctor about any changes in your sex life that may have been caused by your medication and ask about alternative drugs with fewer side effects.

For intercourse, lying side to side with your partner entering from the rear works well if you have hip spasms. This position also allows your partner to stimulate your clitoris with his hands or a vibrator during intercourse. You may need this increased stimulation if you have lost some feeling in your genitals. You and your partner should explore your entire body for other erogenous zones.

Spinal Cord Injury and Sex

A spinal cord injury can be devastating. The loss of movement and feeling in parts of your body can make you afraid that you will never be a sexual person again. Until recently, even doctors thought spinal cord injuries meant the end of sexual pleasure for women. But we now know that a satisfying sex life is possible with all types of spinal cord injury.

First, check your emotions. It is difficult to have a healthy libido if you're depressed and have low self-esteem. You also may have to deal with many physical changes. Paralysis of your upper and/or lower body can make positioning for intercourse difficult. In addition, you may be afraid of incontinence during sex. And the sensitivity of your genitals may have changed since your injury. Don't give up, though. You'll have to make adjustments, but a satisfying sex life is possible with planning, imagination, and a willingness to experiment.

What to Do

Holding and being held by someone you care about can be very sexually satisfying. You and your partner should spend time exploring your body to find areas that give you pleasurable sensations; you may discover how erogenous lips, mouth, neck, ears, and eyelids can be. Stimulating your senses of smell, sight, touch, taste, and hearing during lovemaking will increase the intensity and pleasure of the encounter. Your brain is your largest sex organ, and the world of fantasy can increase your arousal and enjoyment.

If you desire intercourse, use pillows to assist you in positioning your body for optimum pleasure. Try lying on your back with your legs over the side of the bed. Your partner stands, supports his body weight, and enters from above. He can raise and support your legs to change the depth and angle of penetration. You also might try side-to-side as well as the missionary positions. It may make you feel more relaxed and secure if you plan sex after your bladder and bowels have been emptied to decrease the likelihood of an accident.

Masturbation with your fingers or a vibrator may be satisfying. If you have difficulty using your hands, don't be ashamed to ask your partner, a trusted friend, or caretaker to help you position sex toys. Small vibrators can be placed inside your underwear, or a larger vibrator, such as the Hitachi Magic Wand, can be positioned between your legs without difficulty.

Studies have shown that approximately 50 percent of women with spinal cord injury can achieve orgasm through mental imagery or stimulation of erogenous zones—something that was once thought impossible. Your orgasm may take longer to achieve and may be different from what you experienced before your injury, but it can still be exciting.

Stroke and Sex

All aspects of your sexuality may be affected by a stroke. It can impact the way you feel about yourself as a sexual person, and fear of rejection can affect how you relate to your partner. You may feel depressed, anxious, and fearful that sex will cause another stroke. This increased stress can make your libido plummet.

Changes in your body can affect your sexuality. If your muscles are weak or spastic, it may be difficult to have intercourse in the way you were accustomed. The feeling in your genitals also may have changed, making it more difficult to have an orgasm.

What to Do

You don't have to give up an active sex life if you don't want to. Most doctors agree that you can safely resume sexual activity as soon as you feel interested and strong. You and your partner should take the time to explore the many parts of your body to find the areas that are sensitive and turn you on. You may find that some areas that once gave you pleasure have changed—and at the same time you may discover new pleasure points.

The side-by-side rear-entry position may be good if you have weakness on one side or have difficulty spreading your thighs. Lie on your weak side so that you have use of your stronger hand for exploring your partner's body or stimulating your clitoris during intercourse. This position is also good for mutual masturbation, outercourse, and oral sex. If you have decreased genital sensations after your stroke, consider adding a vibrator for more stimulation and variety.

Cancer

The words *it's cancer* can cause instant emotional distress. Anger, confusion, disbelief, anxiety, guilt, and depression are common emotions that people experience after receiving a cancer diagnosis. As you become focused on survival, you may automatically put sex on the back burner. While your desire for sex may decrease, your need for physical closeness may increase. A hug, touch, or caress can give you the emotional support you need, and maintaining intimacy with your partner can help to reduce stress and promote healing. Your partner also may be affected by your diagnosis. Stress and fear of hurting you, of contracting cancer, or of being harmed by the chemotherapy or radiation you may be receiving all can cause a loss of desire or problems with erections. Keep the lines of communication open and discuss your feelings honestly with your partner.

The good news is that most women diagnosed with cancer experience a gradual return of sexual desire. Most couples resume sex within six months of the diagnosis, but some couples may take a year or more. Discuss any concerns you have with your doctor or a qualified sex therapist.

Treatments for cancer may interfere with your desire and enjoyment of sex. The constant stress of frequent hospital and doctor visits for therapy can leave you emotionally drained. Meanwhile, surgery, chemotherapy, and radiation all have the potential to decrease your ability to become aroused and to achieve orgasm. Before we discuss how to rebound sexually from several particular kinds of cancer, let's look at various treatments and their sexual side effects.

Surgery

Surgery for cancer can affect your self-esteem and self-image. If you have to have a breast removed, for instance, you may seek to avoid sex totally for fear that your partner will find the change in your body unattractive. Having your ovaries removed also can be a major downer for your sexuality. Estrogen and androgen levels decrease immediately in women who are not menopausal. Loss of estrogens causes symptoms of menopause, including hot flashes, mood swings, and vaginal dryness. Women who are menopausal prior to surgery will experience a decrease in androgen levels. Loss of androgens may cause decreased libido and difficulty achieving orgasm.

Chemotherapy

Chemotherapy's side effects—nausea, vomiting, weight fluctuations, and fatigue—may dampen your desire for sex. If you lose your hair, it may be difficult for you to view yourself as a sexy and sexual person. Chemotherapy may damage your ovaries, sending you into an early menopause.

Radiation Therapy

It may be difficult to think of sex when you are experiencing the side effects of radiation therapy: fatigue, diarrhea, nausea, skin soreness, and burning. Radiation placed in your vagina can cause it to become swollen and sensitive. As your vagina heals, it can become scarred, stiff, dry, and smaller, making intercourse painful and difficult.

Breast Cancer and Sex

In our culture, women's breasts are a symbol of femininity and sexual attractiveness, and some women and their partners find breast stimulation important for sexual arousal and foreplay. Most women do not notice a change in their sex lives after treatment for breast cancer, but for one-third of women, sexual desire, arousal, and orgasm may decrease. As you recover and begin to feel better, your desire for sex returns; after one year, most women have completely regained their desire.

The primary treatment for breast cancer is surgery, which may mean the removal of the breast (*mastectomy*) or removal of the cancerous lump

Coping with Cancer Treatment Side Effects

Vaginal Dryness

Discuss the safety of estrogen therapy with your doctor. If estrogen is off-limits, vaginal moisturizers such as Lubrin or vitamin E oil may be applied to your vagina three times a week to keep the vagina moist when you are not having sex. Apply a generous amount of water-based lubricants to increase your enjoyment during sex.

Menopausal Symptoms

Surgery, radiation, and chemotherapy can send you into an instant menopause. Loss of estrogen causes your vagina to become dry and decreases your arousal. Without androgen, your desire for sex may decrease and your clitoris may be less sensitive. Discuss therapy with estrogen, androgen, herbs, and other holistic treatments with your doctor.

Vaginal Shortening

Surgery and radiation may cause your vagina to shorten and make sex uncomfortable. Choose positions that enable you to control the depth of penetration of his penis. Lying on your back with your legs straight and close together will effectively lengthen your vagina and increase stimulation of your clitoris.

(*lumpectomy*) and lymph nodes. Some women elect to have a new breast constructed after mastectomy. Changes in the appearance of your breasts may cause feelings of embarrassment and insecurity and may affect your self-image. You may not feel as sexy as you did before surgery, and you may become uncomfortable undressing in front of your partner and having your breasts touched. You also may avoid sexual positions that make it easy to observe your breasts or scars. And your breasts, once sensitive to touch, may feel almost numb after surgery and radiation.

What to Do

Resume sex as soon as you feel comfortable after recovering from surgery. Choose positions that keep your partner's weight off your breasts in the early days of recovery. If changes in your breast make you feel uncomfortable about your appearance, try wearing a sexy bra or negligee during sex. Your body has numerous erogenous zones. Take the time to discover new ones.

Cervical Cancer and Sex

Most cases of cervical cancer are caused by the human papilloma virus, a sexually transmitted infection. With this in mind, many women fear resuming sex after treatment for cervical cancer because they're afraid sex may cause a recurrence. Their partners likewise may fear "catching" cancer from sex. The nature of the diagnosis may make some women feel guilty about their past sexual behavior and view their cervical cancer as punishment. And we all know how guilt can smother the flames of desire.

The treatment for cervical cancer most commonly includes *radical hysterectomy*—removal of the uterus and 25 percent of the vagina—or radiation. Radiation therapy can make your vagina dry, thin, stiff, and almost numb. Sexual intercourse may be painful, and you may experience bleeding and soreness after sex.

What to Do

If your vagina has been shortened by radiation or surgery, choose positions for intercourse that give you control of penetration. The woman-on-top position will enable you to control the depth of penetration. Keeping your legs together while on the bottom will effectively increase the length of your vagina and prevent deep penetration. Be sure to spend more time on foreplay to allow your vagina to lubricate and expand prior to intercourse.

After radiation therapy, your doctor will prescribe dilators to offset the changes in your vagina from radiation. The dilators should be lubricated with either estrogen cream or a water-based lubricant and inserted into your vagina for 15 minutes a day three to four times a week during your recovery from radiation therapy and for years to follow. This will prevent your vagina from becoming narrow, short, and small as it heals. As you become more comfortable, intercourse can substitute for some or all of the dilator sessions. I also recommend a daily massage of the vagina using your fingers and vitamin E oil. Massage stretches the vaginal tissue, prepares it for intercourse, and keeps you in touch with your body. The EROS-CTD, a suction device described later in this book, and Viagra may also improve the blood flow and moisture of your vagina.

Ovarian and Endometrial Cancers and Sex

The primary treatment for ovarian cancer and endometrial cancer is removal of the uterus and ovaries. If you are not menopausal before surgery, your levels of estrogen and androgen drop immediately after surgery, and you are sent into menopause. Hot flashes, mood swings, and vaginal dryness can dampen your desire for sex and cause painful intercourse. Your arousal and orgasms may suffer because of falling androgen levels. Chemotherapy and radiation may cause additional side effects.

What to Do

Estrogen therapy will keep your vagina and vulva moist. If you do not want to use estrogen, use water-based lubricants for sex and vaginal moisturizers three times a week. Discuss with your physician the possibility of testosterone therapy to treat libido and orgasm difficulties.

Vulvar Cancer and Sex

Vulvar cancer is commonly treated by removing part of the vulva. In some cases, a *vulvectomy,* removal of the labia, mons, and a portion, or all, of the clitoris is necessary. The change in the appearance of your vulva may initially affect your self-image and decrease your desire for sex. You may worry that your partner will be turned off by the changes in your sexual anatomy. Side effects of the surgery may include scarring of the opening to your vagina, making intercourse painful, and your vulva may feel numb. Removal of the clitoris may or may not affect your ability to experience orgasm. Despite the physical changes, studies show that after one year, most women with vulvar cancer have returned to an active and satisfying sex life.

What to Do

Resume sex soon after the incisions have healed. A dilator may be used to treat scarring of the vagina, or surgical correction may be necessary. Try using a vibrator on your vulva to stimulate any remaining clitoral tissue. Explore your vagina to find areas of increased sensitivity and pleasure.

Vaginal Cancer and Sex

A large portion of the vagina may be surgically removed, and intercourse may be impossible.

What to Do

Find alternative ways to explore your sexuality. Masturbation, caressing, and oral or anal sex are options.

Other Medical Problems

Back Pain and Sex

Chronic back pain can throw a wrench into your sex life. The muscles of the back are instrumental in pelvic movements. If you're experiencing back pain, you may feel reluctant to have sex for fear that your pain will worsen. But back pain need not spell an end to great sex. With a little ingenuity, you still can have fantastic, satisfying sex. And it may interest you to know that orgasm may relieve back pain for hours.

What to Do

Check with your doctor to be sure your back pain doesn't represent a serious health problem. If your doctor has prescribed an anti-inflammatory medication, such as ibuprofen, naproxen, Vioxx, Celebrex, or aspirin, try taking a dose an hour before sex. A warm shower or bath before sex will help to relax tense back muscles as will an erotic massage with warm oil.

The spoon position can decrease the strain on your back during sex. Sometimes it helps your back if you place a pillow between your legs. You can also try the missionary position with some modifications. Place two firm pillows under your knees to keep them flexed (to help to straighten your back). Your partner should support his entire body weight with his hands or arms as he enters from above. Gentle steady pelvic movements are better for your back than vigorous thrusting movements. You should avoid the woman-on-top position because it may cause you to arch and strain your back.

Irritable Bowel Syndrome and Sex

Irritable bowel syndrome (IBS) is very common in young women. Symptoms include cramping abdominal pain, constipation and/or diarrhea, mucus in your stools, bloating, and gas. Irritable bowel also may cause chronic pelvic pain. Any one of these symptoms can interfere with your ability to have satisfying sex.

The most common sexual complaint of women with IBS is decreased libido. You may also have pain during and just after sex because your bowel, uterus, and ovaries lie very close to one another in your pelvis and share some of the same nerve supply. Pain most commonly occurs with deep vaginal penetration.

What to Do

You can increase your pleasure by choosing positions that decrease the depth of penetration during intercourse. Woman-on-top positions will give you more control, and if you keep your legs straight, penetration will not be as deep. Try gentle rocking movements during intercourse rather than vigorous thrusting to reduce the jarring effect against your bowels.

Avoid eating a heavy meal before sex; it's probably best not to eat anything within two hours of having sex. Stress often aggravates irritable bowel syndrome, so practice relaxation techniques in preparation for lovemaking.

Lung Disease and Sex

Sexual activity increases your body's need for oxygen. Beginning with arousal, your heart rate increases and your breath quickens. Your respiratory rate continues to increase during sex and peaks at orgasm. If you have chronic obstructive lung disease (bronchitis and emphysema) or asthma, this increased exertion may cause breathlessness and fatigue. For a few asthmatics, emotional arousal alone can cause wheezing. And some women have worsening of asthma after orgasm. You may find it difficult to relax and fully enjoy sex when even prolonged kissing can make breathing difficult. If sex causes you to have shortness of breath, wheezing, or coughing, the thought of sex may make you feel anxious and afraid, causing your libido to plummet. Some of the medications you take to help you breathe may impact your sexuality.

What to Do

Using your inhaler and sucking on a cough drop may help to prevent wheezing and coughing during lovemaking. Choose positions that do not place pressure on your chest. Good ones to try are the spoon position, the sitting position facing forward; woman-on-top (allow him to do most of the moving); standing position (you stand and lean, supporting your upper body over the bed as he enters from the rear); and man-on-top (you lie on the bottom with firm pillows propping up your head and chest, and he lies on top and supports his weight with his hands).

Some experts recommend a water bed for sexual intimacy. The gentle rocking motion of the water bed decreases the amount of energy you have to expend during sex. Otherwise, a firm mattress is better than a soft one. Remove all pillows and throws that might interfere with airflow and your ability to breathe.

Let the ease of your breathing dictate the pace of your lovemaking. If you begin to get short of breath or tired, slow down the rhythm or stop for a while. Continue to touch and communicate with your partner and resume sex when you are more energized. You may find that pursing your lips and breathing deeply from your diaphragm before and during sex give you more stamina.

If you need oxygen therapy, you can try using oxygen before beginning sexual activity, or if you need continuous oxygen, tape nasal prongs in place and use a tube extension so the oxygen source does not interfere with your ability to move.

Gyn Problems That Can Affect Sex

Fibroids and Sex

Fibroids are benign, noncancerous tumors that grow in the muscle layer of the uterus. About one-third of all women, and half of African American women have them. These tumors may range in size from that of a pea to larger than a basketball, and you may have one or more of them lodged inside, outside, or within the walls of the uterus. Most women with fibroids have no symptoms or problems, especially if the tumors are small. You might not even know you have them until your doctor discovers that your uterus is enlarged during a routine pelvic examination. An ultrasonogram may be used to confirm the diagnosis. As long as the fibroids don't cause you any discomfort, your gynecologist may recommend no treatment but will watch to see if there are any changes in their size or your symptoms.

Other women may complain of pain, heavy bleeding, constipation, the need to urinate frequently, loss of urine when coughing or jogging, and increased abdominal size as a result of fibroids. These symptoms will probably prompt you and your caregiver to take more action.

How Might Fibroids Affect Your Sex Life?

Most women with fibroids have no problems with sexual performance or enjoyment. Others will have pain and discomfort that interfere with sexual desire and performance. Fibroids may cause a generalized discomfort or the urge to urinate or have a bowel movement as the uterus is forced against the bladder or rectum during intercourse. They may also cause intense cramping pain during orgasm that may last for several hours after intercourse has ended.

Fibroids that are large or located on the bottom part of your uterus may press against the top of your vagina, shortening it and making deep penetration painful and sometimes impossible. Your partner may complain that he can't get all the way into your vagina or that he feels as if he is hitting against something.

Your choice of birth control methods may be limited by large fibroids, which may displace your cervix or change the shape of your vagina so much that it is impossible to snugly fit a diaphragm or cervical cap. Bleeding or pain due to fibroids may be worsened by the use of an IUD. Most studies have found that birth control pills do not cause fibroids to grow and may in fact be used to decrease heavy bleeding in some women. Condoms are a good, safe option.

What to Do

The most common treatment for fibroids is surgery: *myomectomy* (removing only the fibroids) and hysterectomy. A new nonsurgical procedure called *uterine artery embolization* may be used to shrink fibroids and does not appear to affect sexual functioning. You should discuss all of your options with your doctor and be sure to get at least one other opinion.

Choose sexual positions, like the woman-on-top position, that enable you to limit depth of penetration and avoid any painful areas.

Urinating before sex may make you feel more comfortable, and I sometimes recommend taking an anti-inflammatory drug such as ibuprofen one hour before sex to prevent painful intercourse or orgasm.

Fibrocystic Breasts and Sex

Fibrocystic breast changes, most common among women between the ages of thirty and fifty, may cause your breasts to swell and become tender. The discomfort may worsen up to two weeks before and during your period. Since many women (and men) find stimulation of the breasts to be a natural and pleasurable part of sex play, breast tenderness and pain can interfere with sexual enjoyment.

Fibrocystic changes in the breast occur when your breasts respond to your normal fluctuating hormones in an exaggerated manner, becoming tender and swollen. No one knows why some women respond this way and others don't.

What to Do

To ease the discomfort, wear a bra that supports your breasts well—even during sex play. Choose positions that keep pressure off your breasts: Woman-on-top and side-to-side positions work well. You and your partner should avoid stimulating your breasts when they are sensitive.

Caffeine may make tenderness worse, so avoid colas, coffee, chocolate, and even some medications. Some women find taking vitamin E supplements and nonsteroidal anti-inflammatory drugs like ibuprofen to be helpful. If you're taking birth control pills or hormone replacement therapy, changing the type or dose of your medication may help ease breast pain. Ask your doctor about your options.

When Your Treatment Hurts Your Sex Life

Many of the treatments that we use every day for nonsexual medical problems have the potential to wreak havoc on our sex lives. Few of us question our doctors about how prescribed treatments might affect our sex lives—but we should. Here are some of the common surgeries and medications that may affect your sexuality and some suggestions for dealing with them in a sex-positive way.

Surgery That May Affect Your Enjoyment of Sex

Almost any surgical procedure has the potential to affect your sex life, at least for a while. Procedures that involve your vagina, pelvis, and abdomen, in particular, can cause problems with sexual enjoyment. Before undergoing any surgical procedure, it is important to discuss the potential effects on your sex life. Be sure your doctor understands what activities give you pleasure. For instance, if your sexual trigger is your cervix, you will need to discuss whether leaving your cervix intact is a possibility before having a hysterectomy for fibroids. And before leaving the hospital after surgery, be sure to find out when it is safe to resume sex and what, if any, activities to avoid. Few doctors will bring up the topic, so don't be afraid to ask.

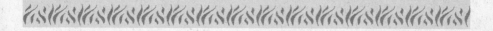

How Infertility May Affect Your Sex Life

Infertility testing can place severe sexual stress on a couple. The need to have sex on demand may lead to a loss of desire and difficulty in arousal and orgasm, and the inability to become pregnant may cause anxiety, depression, and decreased libido. The focus of sex moves from pleasure to procreation. "Making love" is replaced by "making a baby." Spontaneity may be lost, and the pressure to have sex at a specific time, in a specific position, with a specific result can turn sex into a mechanical event. You may experience vaginal dryness and pain with intercourse and find it difficult to reach orgasm.

Men in particular may have a very difficult time. It is not unusual for a young man to have difficulty achieving an erection for the first time when he is told that he must get an erection at a specific time to complete a fertility test. Some men may also find it difficult to ejaculate on demand.

The pressure to perform can kill what is usually an exciting and pleasurable event. Sex becomes stressful more than pleasurable. While trying to conceive my first child, I told my husband, "You don't have to enjoy it. Just deposit the sperm near my cervix."

Talk to your partner about how you feel. Sometimes getting a counselor or therapist involved will make this time more relaxing and comfortable for you both.

Hysterectomy

Hysterectomy is the surgical removal of the uterus and, in most cases, the cervix. It remains one of the most common surgical procedures performed on women. It is a common treatment for fibroids, endometriosis, pelvic pain, and some pelvic cancers. In fact, by the age of sixty, one out of every three women in the United States will have had a hysterectomy, according to some estimates.

The effect of hysterectomy on female sexuality has been controversial, with some studies showing improvement in sexual functioning and others showing deterioration. The majority of women undergoing hysterectomy for benign disease report an improvement in their libido, arousal, and orgasm after surgery. If your uterus is causing pain or excessive bleeding that cannot be controlled, removing it may greatly improve your quality of life and your enjoyment of sex.

However, for approximately 20 percent of women who have had a hysterectomy, sex becomes less desired and enjoyable. For some women, the uterus is important to their femininity and sexual attractiveness. When it is removed, they may suffer decreased self-esteem, depression, loss of libido, and inability to enjoy sex. Removal of the uterus and cervix may shorten and scar the top of the vagina, making sex painful. You may also notice a change in your orgasms if stimulation of your cervix is important in your sexual response. Likewise, if contractions of your uterus play a significant part in the intensity of your orgasms, a hysterectomy may lessen your pleasure.

When a hysterectomy is performed for benign disease, I prefer to leave the cervix (the lower part of the uterus); this is called a *supracervical* hysterectomy. Some studies suggest that this procedure causes less damage to the nerves and blood vessels that run along the cervix and the top of the vagina, so that sexual arousal is not compromised. Also, since the cervix and vagina are not affected, this procedure may not affect orgasms as much as the traditional hysterectomy. If your pap smears have always been normal, the risk of cervical cancer in the cervix that is left behind is very low. With the ability of current technology to detect precancerous changes in the cervix, the possibility of cervical cancer in the future should not be a reason to remove a healthy cervix. You will, however, need to continue to get regular pap smears after surgery.

Removal of the Ovaries

The ovaries produce estrogen, progesterone, and testosterone. Removing the ovaries causes an immediate surgical menopause, causing estrogen levels to plummet and decreasing testosterone levels by 50 percent. Estrogen is what keeps the vagina moist and healthy, so its loss can cause vaginal dryness and reduced engorgement of the vagina and clitoris during arousal. Testosterone is what fuels sexual desire, sensitivity of your genitals, and orgasm. Its loss may cause a decrease in libido, energy, and clitorial sensitivity as well as difficulty achieving orgasm and decreased intensity of orgasm. Discuss estrogen and testosterone replacement therapy with your doctor.

Incontinence Surgery

While most women will notice no change in their sexual response, approximately 20 percent of women who undergo vaginal surgery (vaginal repair) for incontinence of urine complain of problems with sex after surgery. Pain during intercourse and numbness in the vagina are the most common complaints. And some women have lost their ability to have orgasms from stimulation of the G-spot. A similar number of women complain of sexual problems after the "sling" procedures for incontinence—a procedure in which a strip of natural or synthetic material is used to form a "sling" under your urethra to support it. Be sure to discuss your sexual concerns with your doctor prior to surgery.

Ileostomy and Colostomy

Chronic illnesses such as ulcerative colitis and Crohn's disease as well as cancer of the colon are sometimes treated with surgery that leaves you with a *stoma*—an opening between your bowel and abdominal wall created to allow emptying of bowel contents after a portion of your colon is removed. Fears of leakage, odor, or noise can make it difficult for you to relax and enjoy sex. And having an ostomy bag may interfere with your body image and your sense of your self as a sexual person. Vaginal dryness and scar tissue from surgery may make intercourse painful.

Let your partner know your fears. Some women find that wearing a sexy bustier or negligee that covers the ostomy bag and leaves the vulva free makes them more relaxed during sex. Others have found pretty covers for their ostomy bags. Use lubricants and choose positions that allow you to control the depth of penetration during intercourse. Discuss your concerns with your doctor or ostomy nurse.

Medications That May Douse Your Sexual Fire

Of all the potential causes of sexual dysfunction in women, medication is the one most likely to be overlooked. Very few studies have explored the effect of medications on female sexual performance; most have only examined the effect of various drugs on erection and sexual performance in men. Therefore, many doctors are unfamiliar with how even the most common drugs affect the sex lives of women.

Medications can affect your sexual enjoyment either directly or indirectly. And that includes medications that are prescribed by your doctor and those that you buy over the counter at your local pharmacy. Vaginal lubrication, the desire for sex, and the ability to reach orgasm all can be sabotaged by drugs we take every day. For example, antibiotics can cause vaginal yeast infections that make sex painful. Antihistamines that you take for colds and allergy symptoms can make your mouth and vagina dry and cause kissing, intercourse, and oral sex to be less than enjoyable. Some medications, like steroids and some antidepressants, can cause weight gain. If you develop a poor body image because of increasing weight, you may avoid intimacy. Other medications may make you feel tired, weak, dizzy, and too darn miserable to tackle the physical and emotional demands of sex.

There are hundreds of drugs that can affect your sexuality. Remember that every woman is different, and what destroys sex for your best friend may not have any effect on you, and vice versa. The list that follows, however, includes medications that have been shown to have the potential to interfere with your sexual experience.

If you are concerned that a medication you're taking is causing a problem with your sex life, *don't stop taking it,* but do discuss it with your doctor. She or he may be able to change your dose, change the timing of your dosing, or switch you to another drug. Sometimes, adding a second medication will help counter the sexual effects.

Antihypertensives
The majority of antihypertensives—blood pressure medications—cause sexual problems in men. In women, the data are inconclusive. Some stud-

ies show a moderate effect on female sexuality, and others show no effect at all. The list below shows the potential sexual effects of medications used to treat high blood pressure. Keep in mind that hypertension itself can cause problems with desire and arousal.

Diuretics

Most diuretics have the potential to decrease the desire for sex. Hygroton (chlorthalidone) and Hydrodiuril (hydrochlorothiazide) may dampen libido. Aldactone (spironolactone) blocks the effect of androgens (male hormones) and not only may decrease your desire for sex but has been shown to interfere with orgasm in some women. Lasix has few or no effects on sexual performance in women.

Beta-Blockers

Beta-blockers, including Inderal (propranolol), Tenormin (atenolol), Lopressor (metoprolol), and Corgard (nadolol), increase your levels of serotonin, which decreases your sex drive. Your ability to reach orgasm also may be slowed or halted. Some women have complained of loss of libido, weakness, fatigue, and depression while taking these drugs.

Others

- Reserpine can cause depression, decreased libido, and decreased arousal.

- Aldomet (methyldopa) increases your prolactin level, which may decrease your desire for sex and make it harder to reach orgasm.

- Ismelin (guanethidine) may decrease your libido and block your orgasm.

- Catapres (clonidine) may have a sedative effect, killing your desire for sex. It also may interfere with your arousal.

- ACE inhibitors—Capoten (captopril), Vasotec (enalapril), Accupril (quinapril)—and calcium channel–blockers—Norvasc (amlodipine), Cardizem (diltiazem), Calan (verapamil)—appear to have no effect on sexual performance.

Antidepressants

Many women experiencing depression complain of problems with sexual performance. It is sometimes difficult to determine whether the problems with desire and arousal are caused by depression or by the medications prescribed to treat it. On the other hand, successful treatment for depression may restore desire and arousal.

Tricyclic Antidepressants

Drugs in this category include Elavil (amitriptyline), Tofranil (imipramine), Pamelor (nortriptyline), Vivactil (protriptyline), and Anafranil (clomipramine). Decreased libido and difficulty achieving orgasms are side effects common to all of these. Pain during orgasm is a rare side effect of some drugs in this class. If you're taking tricyclic antidepressants, intercourse may become painful due to increased dryness of your vagina, and dry mouth may interfere with your enjoyment of oral sex and kissing. Though you may notice some of these problems when starting treatment, the side effects may resolve after several months.

Interestingly, some women experience an increase in sexual desire while taking Tofranil, and a rare side effect of Anafranil is spontaneous orgasms while yawning.

Monoamine Oxidase Inhibitors

Marplan (isocarboxazid), Nardil (phenelzine) and Parnate (tranylcypromine) may depress the libido and cause difficulty achieving orgasm.

Selective Serotonin Reuptake Inhibitors (SSRIs)

Drugs in this class, including Prozac (fluoxetine), Zoloft (sertraline), Paxil (paroxetine), Effexor (venlafaxine), and Luvox (fluvoxamine), commonly depress the libido and cause difficulty achieving orgasm. Having a sexual problem with one SSRI, however, does not mean you will have a problem with another. And problems with desire and orgasm may resolve over time while continuing the same medication. A few women have found that their arousal and orgasms actually improved while taking selective serotonin reuptake inhibitors.

If you have problems with orgasm, your doctor may suggest "drug holidays." Discontinuing the medication on the weekend may boost your libido and your ability to have orgasms without affecting your depression. *Do not stop or change your medication schedule without the direction of your doctor.* Some doctors will add another medication to your regimen to improve your sex life. Yohimbine and Viagra are two medications that have been shown to decrease the sexual side effects of drugs in this class. Two antidepressants, Wellbutrin (bupropion) and Desyrel (trazodone), have been shown to improve sexual desire. Serzone (nefazodone) does not appear to have sexual side effects.

Antianxiety/Sedatives

Anxiety is a common cause of sexual dysfunction. Often, reducing anxiety will help you to relax and enjoy sex. In high doses, however, these medications may decrease your desire for sex and your ability to become aroused. One such drug, Buspar (buspirone), may potentially improve your sex drive and orgasm.

Benzodiazepines

Xanax (alprazolam), Librium (chlordiazepoxide), Klonopin (clonazepam), Valium (diazepam), and Ativan (lorazepam) are examples of drugs in this class. All may decrease desire and interfere with orgasms when used for long periods of time.

Contraceptives
Birth Control Pills (Oral Contraceptives)

Most women beginning to take birth control pills will experience an increase in their libido. Free from the fear of pregnancy, you may find that your desire for sex increases. Some women, however, experience a decline in their libido after taking the pill for several months or years that is possibly due to the decrease in free testosterone that occurs when taking the pill. Some pills have more of an effect on your testosterone level than others. So changing the type of pill you take will sometimes improve your desire. Pills containing 20 mcg of estrogen and those containing the progesterone levonorgestrel (found in Lo-Ovral, Nordette, Levlen, Levlite) may have less of a depressive effect on your libido.

Oral contraceptives may cause vaginal dryness that leads to pain with intercourse, and while on the pill some women develop depression—a surefire libido buster.

Progesterone Shots and Implants

Depo-provera and Norplant use progesterone hormone to prevent pregnancy. While most women experience no change in their enjoyment of sex while using progesterone for contraception, some women suffer a decline in their sexual desire and pleasure. Progesterone may dampen sensations in your pelvis and interfere with orgasm. Your desire for sex may decline if you experience irregular bleeding, mood swings, and weight gain—common progesterone side effects.

Other Medications

- Tagament (cimetidine), which is used to decrease stomach acid, blocks histamine and, since histamine plays a part in orgasms, may make the achievement of orgasm more difficult. Cimetidine also may decrease libido.

- Nolvadex (tamoxifen), which is used in the treatment of breast cancer, may cause either vaginal dryness or excessive lubrication and has been shown to decrease libido in some women. Most women, however, experience no change in their desire or enjoyment of sex while taking tamoxifen.

- Pondimin (fenfluramine), which is used for weight loss, has caused increased desire and arousal in some women. It's not clear whether it is the weight loss or the drug itself that causes the libido boost.

- Dilantin (phenytoin), which is used to treat seizure disorders, causes an increase in prolactin levels. With prolonged use, it may decrease libido.

- Phenobarbital, which is used in seizure disorders, may decrease sexual desire.

Chapter 20

Psychological and Emotional Issues

Sometimes you may experience problems with sex that have nothing to do with illness or any kind of physical challenge. Sex is complicated—both physically and mentally. For women, the mental and emotional side often far outweighs the physical side of the sexual experience. Let's look at some of the common psychological and emotional issues that may extinguish your sexual fire—or his.

Psychological Issues

Depression

It may be difficult to think of sexual pleasure when you're depressed. In fact, a loss of sexual desire may be one of the first signs of depression.

More than half of women suffering from depression complain of a decline in desire, arousal, or orgasm. Other signs of depression include difficulty sleeping, a pessimistic outlook, difficulty concentrating, loss of pleasure in life, and low self-esteem.

Depression is very common in women. If you are depressed, get help. Depression is a medical problem in much the same way that diabetes and high blood pressure are medical problems. Often when the depression is treated, sexual desire and enjoyment are restored.

Some of the medications used to treat depression may themselves cause sexual problems. Fortunately, as discussed in the previous chapter, there are options.

Body Image

The way you feel about your body directly affects your sexuality. A negative body image, or the feeling that you are not sexually attractive, can make you shy away from sex and hamper your ability to relax and enjoy the ride. If you feel insecure, distracted, and anxious, sex may become mechanical and unsatisfying.

When you worry about the way you look during sex, you avoid positions that make it easier for your partner to see the body part that you find least attractive. You concentrate on moving your lover's hands away from areas of concern like "fat thighs" or "sagging breasts" instead of on the pleasurable sensations of sex. You might insist on having the covers on and the lights off. Perhaps even romantic candlelight is forbidden. You may worry constantly that your lover will notice that you don't have the body of a Victoria's Secret model. Girls, believe me, if you have gotten to the point of having sex with a man, it is highly unlikely that he is going to sabotage his pleasure by worrying about your mid-rib bulge.

Learning to accept your body the way it is will go a long way in improving your sexual satisfaction. You will gain the self-esteem and confidence you need to be seductive, sensual, and in command of your sexual experience. Begin by practicing a little self-love. By that, I mean show yourself how much you love and appreciate the woman you are every day. Start each day with an affirmation—a simple statement that expresses something good and wonderful about yourself. Remember, you can be sexy at any age and alluring at any weight. It's all about how you feel within.

Stress

We all lead stressful lives. As women, we take on the responsibility of making sure that everyone around us is well taken care of and content. To that end, we often find ourselves juggling many roles: mother, housekeeper, laundress, employee/employer, chauffeur for the kids, tutor, cook, friend, daughter, wife, and last and sometimes least, lover. When it comes time for lovemaking, you may be just too darn tired! Superwoman is a myth!

You can begin to tackle your stress by setting priorities. Make a list of your daily tasks and ask others for help. Carve out a few minutes every day for meditation, relaxation, and breathing. A great book to read for guidance is *Self-Nurture* by Alice D. Domar, Ph.D.

Childhood Physical or Sexual Abuse

Childhood abuse can cause feelings of guilt, anger, shame, and depression that have a catastrophic effect on your ability to have healthy sexual relationships. Women who have been abused commonly experience decreased sexual desire and pain with sex as well as problems with arousal and orgasm. Beverly Engel, author of *Raising Your Sexual Self-Esteem*, states that women who were abused as children may suffer from self-hatred, have a poor body image, and find it difficult to express sexual feelings.

If you have been abused, it is important to see a therapist. Working through your feelings, conscious and unconscious, will help you to develop a healthy sense of self and a more satisfying sex life.

Negative Childhood Messages

"Sex is bad, dirty, sinful."

"Sex is dangerous. Don't let boys touch you."

"Touching yourself 'down there' is bad."

"Good girls don't."

"Women don't enjoy sex."

These are but a few of the messages that women sometimes hear as little girls. The messages you receive as a child from religious teaching, your parents, and society may affect your sexual self-esteem as an adult. Negative messages about your body, genitals, masturbation, homosexuality, men, and sex can cause guilt, shame, and fear that last a lifetime and make it difficult to enjoy sex. The foundation for your sexuality is laid long before you are able to enjoy it.

Sit down and make a list of all of the negative sexual messages that you received as a child. Now change each statement from a negative to a positive one. For example, "Women don't enjoy sex" becomes "I have a right to sexual pleasure." Every time one of those negatives messages enters your mind, flip it over to the positive side.

Partner Issues

He Is Not in the Mood

It's a myth that men are always ready and willing to have sex. Women often assume that if a man doesn't get an automatic erection, he lacks interest. Like women, men may be affected by fatigue, stress, sleep deprivation, mood swings, and performance anxiety. Medical problems and medications can affect his performance and libido as well.

For many men, aging brings on a loss of desire. In the middle-age years (forty to fifty), almost one in five men complains of decreased desire, according to the NHSLS survey. In my practice, the decreased desire of male partners is one of the most common complaints of women in their forties. Often as a woman is coming into her own sexually, her partner is winding down. When our men decrease the frequency of sexual initiation or turn down our requests for lovemaking, we may feel rejected and depressed. We assume that something is wrong with us and that he doesn't love us or find us attractive. We may even fear that someone else is stoking his fire. His lowered libido may directly affect our self-esteem. We may even begin to avoid sex for fear of rejection. Communication with your partner is the key. Let him know your fears and desires.

Erectile Dysfunction (ED)

Almost every man will have at least one experience during which he is unable to achieve or maintain an erection long enough to complete sexual intercourse. The cause can be as simple as having too much to drink or feeling exhausted. The first time he is unable to become erect or maintain his erection, both of you may feel devastated. He may worry that he has lost the ability forever, and you may worry that he no longer finds you attractive. You may even begin to doubt your sexual technique.

Easy, automatic, spontaneous erections begin to decrease in the mid-thirties for many men. The initial reactions of most are fear and anxiety. Your partner may become overly concerned and worried about his erections—and those fears will only interfere further with his ability to respond.

Many women, and men, are unaware of the fact that as men age they need stimulation of the penis as well as sexual thoughts to get a good erection. A picture of an attractive woman may have done the trick at age twenty, but he may need a little stroking of your hand or lips in addition to the picture to move things along at age forty.

There are many causes of ED. Alcohol, drugs, and stress can all cause a temporary inability to become erect. Medications and medical problems such as diabetes, cardiovascular disease, hypertension, kidney disease, prostate surgery, and spinal cord injury may cause erectile dysfunction.

A urologist can help your partner decide which treatment is best, based on the cause of his dysfunction. Treatment options include self-injections of medications directly into the penis, a suppository containing prostaglandin that is placed in his urethra, vacuum devices that force blood into the penis to make it erect, and penile implants. The newest treatment for ED is Viagra, a pill that works by inducing smooth-muscle relaxation and increasing blood flow to the penis to cause an erection.

Premature Ejaculation

Premature ejaculation is the most common male sexual problem. According to the NHSLS survey, 21 percent of men complained of premature ejaculation. A man is said to have premature ejaculation if he repeatedly reaches orgasm or ejaculates before, on, or shortly after penetration, and if the situation is causing him personal distress. Premature ejaculation commonly causes loss of self-esteem, embarrassment, and performance anxiety. Some men develop erectile dysfunction or may avoid sex altogether. If intercourse is important to you, his inability to perform may cause you to become frustrated or disappointed. On the other hand, you may avoid any intimate contact to spare him feelings of inadequacy.

A combination of medical treatment and sex therapy may be helpful in reversing premature ejaculation. Two techniques suggested by sex therapists are the *squeeze technique* and the *stop-start technique*.

Squeeze Technique

Manually or orally stimulate your partner until he is close to ejaculation. You then stop and squeeze the head of his penis (at the level of the frenulum) firmly between your thumb and first two fingers until his urge to come has subsided. He may lose his erection partially but will regain it with resumption of oral or manual stimulation. You repeat these steps four or five times before you allow him to ejaculate. You can practice this same technique during intercourse, but some men find it more difficult to maintain control.

Stop-Start Technique

Manually or orally stimulate your partner. When he gets close to ejaculation, you stop all contact with his penis until his urge to ejaculate has passed. Then resume stimulation. Repeat four or five times before allowing him to ejaculate.

Charles and Caroline Muir, authors of *Tantra: The Art of Conscious Loving,* describe another technique to delay ejaculation, called *the pull,* that can be used during intercourse. When your partner feels close to ejaculation, either you or he gently squeezes and pulls down on the top of his scrotum (right where the scrotum and the penis meet, not the testicles). Hold the squeeze until the urge to ejaculate passes, which usually takes 10–30 seconds, then resume intercourse.

For some men, wearing a condom reduces sensitivity enough to allow them sufficient control of ejaculation. Antidepressants, particularly the selective serotonin reuptake inhibitors (SSRIs), may be effective in treating premature ejaculation.

Male Orgasmic Disorder

In my practice, I have seen numerous women who have been extremely distressed by their partner's inability to ejaculate during intercourse. Each woman expressed doubts about her desirability, attractiveness, and sexual technique. They questioned whether their partners cared for them and felt inadequate and depressed. And because they constantly monitored the response of their partners, they were unable to relax and enjoy their sexual experiences. This disorder is rarely discussed, yet in the NHSLS approximately 8 percent of men had experienced the inability to ejaculate at least some of the time.

Causes of male orgasmic disorder include alcohol, medications, neurological disorders, performance anxiety, past trauma, and fear of causing a pregnancy. Collaboration between a urologist and psychologist or sex therapist is the most effective therapy.

Relationship Issues

As a gynecologist who believes sexual health is a major part of general health and happiness, I have heard many complaints from women about relationship issues that affect their sexuality. In the past twenty years, the concerns voiced have not changed and appear to be universal. A few of the most common are listed below.

Lack of Tenderness

The most common relationship complaint I hear is the lack of tenderness and intimacy. Women desire more holding, touching, caressing, romancing, and hugging. When intimacy is lacking, you may not feel loved, appreciated, desired, and secure enough to relax and enjoy sex.

For many men, affection and sex are synonymous. These men may only show affection when it leads to sex. Women may begin to avoid any physical contact with their partners because, for some men, touching means you are ready for sex, when all you may want is a hug or to be held close.

One sex therapist suggests that you "give what you want to get." Meaning, give your partner a hug or cuddle and let him know how good that makes you feel. You might say, "I love being able to hug you even though we're not having sex."

Not Enough Foreplay

Most women need and desire more foreplay than men to become sufficiently aroused before intercourse. When sex begins and ends according to his erection, you may feel left out. Many women also desire continued affection, such as snuggling, when intercourse is over. Talk honestly with your partner about your sexual needs and desires. You might clue him in by saying something like: "Honey, I love touching, hugging, and kissing that gorgeous body of yours before we have sex."

Problems with His Technique

Sometimes his technique is not exactly compatible with your sexual needs or desires, and you're probably reluctant to say anything because you don't want to hurt his feelings. Remember, your mate was not born knowing exactly how to satisfy you sexually. Every woman is different. If he can't find your clitoris or his touch isn't just right for you, then you must take responsibility for your own sexual pleasure. Taking responsibility means communicating with your partner to let him know what turns you on.

Boredom

When you have been with your partner for a while, it's easy to get into a sexual routine where you follow the same sexual script with each encounter: Sex occurs at the same time and the same place, and begins and ends the same way.

Imagine eating your favorite meal prepared the same way, with the same spices, and served on the same plate day after day and year after year. Soon you would no longer salivate when it was placed in front of you, and eventually you would lose all desire for it. Variety is indeed the spice of life. You may want to refer to Chapter 4 for suggestions of ways to spice up your love life.

Unrealistic Expectations

Do you remember what it was like when you first fell in love with your mate? Early in your relationship you may have had palpitations just thinking about your lover. His touch, smell, and the sound of his voice were enough to awaken your desire. The hormones and chemicals of love worked their magic and every time you made love, firecrackers went off, bombs exploded, and all was well with the world. It doesn't get any better than that, but such infatuation doesn't last forever. The relationship settles down into one that is more gentle and nurturing, which happens for most couples somewhere between one year and two and a half years. When that intense chemistry wears off, you may wake up and say to yourself, "I am in bed with *who*?" You may wonder if you have "fallen out of love" with your partner. You may be puzzled and miss the excitement and mystery of the earlier days of the relationship.

There are ways to keep the excitement going in your relationship. It doesn't have to become stale; but it may be unrealistic to expect it to remain exactly the same as it was in the early days of courtship. It is important to realize you're not alone. Relationships change and evolve over time, and change doesn't have to be bad.

The frequency of sex decreases for most couples in the first several years of life together. For some couples, frequency decreases by half in the first year. Experts describe a "honeymoon period" early in the relationship, but after living together for a period of time sex may become routine, the excitement wears off, and the frequency of sex drops off. Work schedules and having children—which often means a loss of privacy and private time as a couple—all add to the dip in lovemaking. If you are not expecting this change and are surprised by it, you may assume there's a problem with the relationship. You may be hurt, confused, and frustrated. You may fear that your partner no longer loves you and worry that the rest of your years together will be unsatisfying.

Sex may not be the way it appears in the movies or romance novels, and it may not be fabulous, passionate, and over-the-top every time. If you are expecting it to be, you may be setting yourself up for disappointment and frustration. My advice is to cultivate more realistic expectations, use some of the techniques suggested in Chapter 4, and always keep the lines of communication open.

Performance Anxiety: Pressure to Perform

Many women feel an intense need to have an orgasm to please their partners, and some men feel responsible for a woman's orgasm. Your partner may view sex as incomplete and unsatisfying unless you achieve orgasm, and he may regard your lack of orgasm as a personal failure. He may begin to doubt his technique as a lover, and making you achieve orgasm may become his mission. In turn, you may feel inadequate and dysfunctional. What should be a pleasurable experience becomes a chore filled with stress.

The National Health and Social Life Survey showed that only 29 percent of women always have orgasm during sex with their partners. Talk with your partner and let him know your feelings about orgasm. Sex is about more than achieving orgasm. It is not a contest or competition. Trying to force or will an orgasm is a sure way to prevent it from happening.

Treating Sexual Problems

Sex Therapy

When your sex life is not what you want it to be, sex therapy can be just what you need to get it back on track or make it better than ever. Even when your problems appear to be purely medical, there are often psychological or relationship issues as well.

Despite the obvious benefits of seeing a sex therapist, I often have problems convincing women or couples to consult with one. Even in New York City, where seeing a therapist of some sort seems as common as buying a cup of coffee in the morning, people are often reluctant to visit a sex therapist. Speaking to a stranger about something as private and intimate as the details of your sex life can be frightening or embarrassing. You may fear being seen as abnormal, weak, perverted, or crazy. Sexual health and enjoyment are important to your quality of life, and sexual problems are common. There is no reason to be embarrassed.

Sex therapists can be viewed as "sex detectives" who can help you identify problems and can make suggestions to help restore sexual health. Often only one to five visits are necessary to get your sex life humming, but more complicated and deep-seated issues may take longer to sort out and work through.

A good therapist is trained to educate you about sex and to motivate you to achieve the healthiest, most satisfying sexual experiences possible. When choosing a sex therapist, make sure she/he is certified by an entity such as the American Academy of Clinical Sexologists or the American Association of Sex Educators, Counselors and Therapists. Your doctor may be able to make a recommendation.

Testosterone

Testosterone is the hormone responsible for your sex drive as well as feelings of assertiveness and aggression. It is also responsible for the sensitivity of your nipples and genitals. As you age, your level of testosterone decreases, and by the time you reach forty, your testosterone level may have decreased to half of what it was when you were twenty.

Before menopause most of your testosterone is produced by your ovaries and a smaller amount by your adrenal glands. After menopause your ovaries continue to produce testosterone, though the amount decreases by half. Testosterone levels may also be decreased by surgery to remove your ovaries, by radiation, or by chemotherapy. Sometimes the cause of low testosterone is unknown.

Most of the testosterone in your body is bound to sex hormone–binding globulins. The remainder is free in your blood, and it is this free testosterone that is active. Your free testosterone may decrease while taking estrogen or birth control pills.

What Happens When Your Testosterone Level Is Low

Your doctor can determine your level of total and free testosterone by doing blood tests. Low testosterone may cause a loss of desire for sex, decreased arousal, and a decline in the incidence or intensity of your orgasms. You may notice that you don't have sexual thoughts or dreams and you never feel "horny." Your energy and sense of well-being may be low.

Libido Boosters

Ten Steps to Spice Up Your Love Life

Make sexual dates with each other. It is a myth that sex should be natural and spontaneous. Spontaneous sex can be overrated. And besides, planned sex is better than no sex. Anticipation of the date can be exciting and arousing. Plan little surprises for each other. For a hot sex date, make a reservation for lunch in a hotel and order room service. A couple of hours in a hotel in the middle of the day with your partner can feel enticingly naughty.

Plan nonsexual couple time together. Given your busy schedule, you may be limited to only a few hours per week. It's the quality of the time that is most important. Plan to spend the time talking and getting to really know each other. Find out his favorite color, what music he is listening to on the way to work, what he eats for lunch, what makes him laugh. During this couple time, complaining, criticizing each other, and discussing bills or the children are not allowed.

For one week, do something romantic every day. Leave a love note in his briefcase, in his lunch box, on the bathroom mirror, on the front seat of his car, or in his coat pocket. Call him midday just to say you were thinking of him and his gorgeous body. Send him an erotic e-mail.

Share a bubble bath or shower together with an aromatic gel. Don't forget the candles, aromatherapy, mood music, and perhaps a small glass of champagne (not too much!).

Talk sexy to each other. Tell him all the things he does that drive you wild. Flirt like you did in the old days. Give cute names to your most intimate body parts.

continued

〰 **Spend an evening pleasuring each other.** Take turns stroking, rubbing, massaging, and caressing each other all over. First lie on your stomach and then your back. Communicate and let each other know what feels good. But skip the breasts and genitals this time.

〰 **Laugh together.** See a comedy show or funny movie, tell each other jokes, or do something silly like wrapping yourself in holiday paper and placing a big red bow on your head. Shared laughter can be oh so erotic.

〰 **Make sexual requests of each other.** Requests, not demands. For instance, "Honey, I just love it when you smear my nipples with raspberry jam and lick it off. Can we try that tonight?"

〰 **Try a new sex toy.** Have fun choosing just the right one from an erotic catalog or Internet site. Better yet, visit a local female-oriented sex shop together. Just think how much you'll laugh together during that field trip!

〰 **Take a romantic weekend trip to a bed-and-breakfast inn.** No kids allowed! Plan it in advance. Look forward to it. If a trip does not fit into your budget, send the children to their grandparents or a friend's home for the evening to allow you to have private sensuous time together.

If you and your mate have been disconnected for some time, you may not feel motivated to try any of these tips. It may feel unnatural or uncomfortable. That's a normal reaction. Take one small step at a time. Read the list together and try to find one thing that feels comfortable for both of you. And don't be afraid to discuss your concerns with a professional counselor.

Your vagina, clitoris, and nipples may be less sensitive; it may take longer to become aroused; and you may have difficulty achieving orgasms. Some women say they feel sexually "numb."

Treatment with Testosterone

There are no FDA-approved testosterone supplements for the treatment of sexual dysfunction in women in the United States, and testosterone therapy is somewhat controversial. Methyltestosterone combined
with estrogen (Estratest) has been approved for the treatment of hot flashes
that do not respond to estrogen alone and can be used in postmenopausal
women with diminished desire.

Your doctor, however, may prescribe (off-label) smaller doses of testosterone supplements that have been designated for use in men. Compound-
ing pharmacies also produce testosterone based on a doctor's prescription.

The following forms of testosterone are made for men but may be used
(with your doctor's instructions) by women with low testosterone levels.

- *Androgel* is a colorless topical gel that provides sustained release
  of testosterone. Some doctors have found that, if a woman uses
  only a fraction of the gel packet prescribed for men, there is an
  increase in desire and sexual response without significant side
  effects.

- *Oral methyltestosterone* has been used in small doses (0.25–1 mg per
  day) with some success in women.

- *Testosterone patches* are made for men and are currently being in-
  vestigated for use in women. Some doctors recommend cutting
  the patches into smaller pieces for female use. A smaller patch
  for women is expected in the future.

- *Testosterone pellets* that can be implanted under your skin are available in some countries.

- *Testosterone injections* are given most commonly once every three
  months. A fraction of the dose used for men may be given
  to women.

Potential Side Effects of Testosterone Therapy

Most of the side effects of testosterone therapy occur when high doses
of testosterone are administered for a prolonged period. Acne, facial hair,

weight gain, deepening of your voice, and increased feelings of aggression have been described. Most side effects are reversed when the medication is discontinued. Some women may have enlargement of the clitoris that is not reversible. An enlarged clitoris may be uncomfortable but is not harmful. High doses of testosterone may cause liver damage and decreased good (HDL) cholesterol. *Women who may become pregnant should not use testosterone because of the harm it may cause a developing fetus.*

Testosterone therapy may not help if your level of testosterone is within the normal range for women. And even some women with low levels do not experience an increase in their desire or enjoyment of sex after starting testosterone therapy. Studies of the long-term safety of testosterone therapy are incomplete. For these reasons, the American College of Obstetrics and Gynecology urges caution in the use of testosterone therapy for female sexual dysfunction; it also recommends low doses and close monitoring of side effects.

Viagra

Viagra was developed to treat erectile dysfunction in men. Viagra, taken one hour before sex, dilates blood vessels, increases blood flow, and causes the penis to become erect. Since increased blood flow is necessary for erection of the clitoris and lubrication of the vagina, one would expect Viagra to have a similar sex-enhancing effect in women. However, the jury is still out concerning the effect of Viagra on female sexual problems. Some researchers have found no improvement in sexual function in women, while others have found a significant improvement in the arousal and orgasms of women taking Viagra. Viagra has been found to be effective in improving arousal and orgasms in women who are taking antidepressants, and I have used it with success to improve the arousal of menopausal women.

Side effects of Viagra include headaches, nausea, abnormal vision, flushing, and digestion problems.

ProSensual

ProSensual is a lubricant that is described as a topical sexual stimulant for women. The ingredients are based on writings in the Kama Sutra and

include a combination of natural oils. Most women describe a warm tingling sensation after applying ProSensual.

Arginmax

Arginmax is an herbal supplement containing ginseng, L-arginine, ginkgo,
damiana, vitamins, and minerals. A study conducted at Stanford University School of Medicine showed that Arginmax increases desire, sexual
frequency, and satisfaction in women.

EROS-CTD

I must admit I was skeptical when I was first introduced to this device.
The thought of using a machine to increase my arousal was not appealing,
but this device really works, and it is well worth the hefty price tag.

The EROS-Clitoral Therapy Device (CTD) is the only device approved
by the FDA for the treatment of female sexual dysfunction. It is a small,
battery-operated vacuum device that fits comfortably in your hand. It has
a small, soft cup that is placed over your clitoris. When you turn it on, it
produces a gentle suction that increases the blood flow to your clitoris,
vulva, and vagina. Your clitoris becomes erect, and vaginal lubrication improves.

You can use the device before sexual intercourse to increase arousal
and sensations, or you may use it alone. It is fun and exciting, but it is not
a sex toy. EROS-CTD is a therapeutic device and is only available by prescription from your doctor. Over time, it may help the blood vessels that
supply your clitoris to work better. It has potential benefit for women who
have problems with arousal, such as those who have had a hysterectomy,
who are postmenopausal, and who have had pelvic radiation. Even women
without sexual problems may achieve increased sensations and orgasms
after using EROS-CTD.

I recommend daily use for a period of several weeks to increase blood
flow to your genitals. Begin with 5 minutes and gradually increase to 15
minutes of daily use. Begin with the lowest vacuum setting, and as you become more comfortable with the device, you can increase the strength of
the suction. Frequent use of the device improves arousal, lubrication, sensitivity, and orgasms in many women.

Erotica

Erotic videos may be educational as well as arousing. New female-sensitive videos, some produced by women, show women in a positive rather than a demeaning light. Erotic videos can increase your arousal, introduce you to new sexual techniques, and increase sexual desire. Erotic videos can also be used as a lead-in to conversations between you and your partner about sex.

Most female-oriented sex shops sell a variety of erotic videos and books. My favorite Internet sites for erotica are www.royalle.com (Candida Royalle's Femme), www.goodvibes.com (Good Vibrations), www.evesgarden.com (Eve's Garden), and www.IntimacyInstitute.com (Sinclair Intimacy Institute).

Sleep and Your Sexuality

We need to be fired up to best accomplish life's basics,
the four F's: foraging, feeding, fighting and fooling
around.

—Dr. William C. Dement
The Promise of Sleep

While You Were Sleeping . . .

While you sleep, your vagina experiences multiple episodes of increased blood flow, engorgement, and lubrication. These episodes are the equivalent of the erections that all men get during REM sleep (the dreaming stage of sleep). No, it doesn't mean that your dreams are erotic or sexual. Like "wet dreams" in men, some women have orgasms while sleeping.

Sleep is important to our health, happiness, and sexuality. Yet most of us are sleep deprived. Inadequate sleep can cause physical and mental exhaustion and decrease your motivation for and enjoyment of sex. It can make you moody, irritable, stressed, and depressed. You have more aches, pains, and discomforts and less extra energy for sex play.

According to Dr. Dement, the average person needs one hour of sleep for every two that they are awake. That means most people need eight hours of sleep every night. Of course, some people will need more and others less. If you feel sleepy, tired, or drowsy during the daytime, you are probably behind in sleep. Learn what your sleep requirements are and work to acquire an adequate amount of sleep every day.

Sleep replenishes the excitatory neurotransmitters in your brain—norepinephrine and dopamine—which increase your motivation and desire for sex as well as your arousal. Sufficient sleep gives you greater energy and vitality. It boosts your desire to fool around as well as your ability to respond to pleasurable sensations.

We all have peaks and valleys in alertness during the day. Try to schedule sex for the hours when you are most energetic. If you prefer bedtime sex and tend to run out of steam in the evening, consider a nap in the afternoon to rev up for a marathon session of lovemaking later.

Chapter 21

When Sex
Is a Pain

When we speak of "hot sex," we usually don't mean it literally. But sex can indeed get hot and painful. And nothing kills a night of sensuous sex like pain, unless, of course, that's what turns you on.

We all have discomfort during or after sex once in a while. For instance, it may be uncomfortable to have intercourse during the middle of your menstrual cycle when you're ovulating. During this time, the ovaries are slightly swollen and tender. If your partner's penis strikes an ovary during intercourse, you may feel sharp pain. Changing your position to decrease the depth of penetration may be all you need to do to avoid further discomfort. You may feel similar discomfort immediately before, during, or after your period. Also, when you have intercourse for the very first time, or for the first time in a while, you may have some discomfort or pain. In fact, it may be the expectation of pain that many women have in these situations that makes the pain worse.

If pain is severe and recurrent, it can make it almost impossible for you to relax and enjoy sex. Your desire for sex may plummet, you may have problems becoming aroused, and achieving orgasm may become more difficult. Pain may occur when your vulva is touched, massaged, or stimulated; when you engage in oral sex; when you attempt penetration with a penis, finger, or sex toy; or when your partner is thrusting deeply into your vagina with a penis, finger, or sex toy.

To help your doctor determine the cause of your pain during sex, answer the following questions and take them to your doctor's visit.

彡 Do you find being touched, penetration of your vagina, or deep thrusting painful?

彡 Is the pain sharp, dull, burning, or stabbing?

彡 Is the pain mild or severe?

彡 Is the pain localized in one spot, or does it affect a larger area?

彡 Do you feel the pain in your vagina or deep inside your pelvis?

彡 Do you get the pain every time you have sex?

彡 Does the pain continue after sex?

彡 Does the pain occur only intermittently during the month?

彡 Does changing positions alleviate the pain?

彡 As intercourse continues, does the pain increase or decrease?

彡 How long have you had problems with pain during sex?

Painful sex is common, occurring in approximately 15 percent of women, according to the National Health and Social Life Survey. Just because pain is common does not mean you should grit your teeth and bear it. I see women daily who continue having sex even though it is extremely painful. One woman said she bites down on a pillow while having sex to keep herself from screaming. You won't get any badges or medals for suffering an injury obtained "in the line of duty." Don't be a martyr. Sex should be a mutually enjoyable experience. If you are having pain and a simple change of position does not take it away, or the pain is severe, stop. Let your partner know you are uncomfortable. Find nonpainful ways to express your sexuality—like cuddling, kissing, massaging, and caressing—until you can see a doctor.

Pain During Stimulation of Your Vulva

If your vulva is irritated or inflamed, merely touching it can be uncomfortable. It may be difficult to find pleasure in masturbation, genital massage, or oral sex. There can be a number of reasons for this kind of pain.

Infections
Infections with bacteria, trichomonas, yeast, herpes, and genital warts can cause swelling, soreness, and pain when your vulva is touched or massaged.

Irritants
Allergic reactions to spermicides, condoms, soaps, detergents, perfumes, or hygiene sprays can cause the skin of your vulva to become inflamed and irritated.

Dermatitis
Any condition that causes inflammation of the skin may make touching and rubbing your vulva uncomfortable. The most common are eczema, lichen sclerosus, psoriasis, and folliculitis (infections at the base of strands of hair).

Vulvodynia

Vulvodynia is a condition that causes constant burning of the vulva. If severe, it may be difficult to wear certain clothing or to sit for long periods of time. One type of vulvodynia is thought to be caused by problems with the nerves in the vulva. These nerves, usually silent, begin to transmit pain signals to your brain either spontaneously or when your vulva is touched. You may find it difficult or impossible to enjoy manual stimulation, oral sex, or intercourse because of the pain. Tricyclic antidepressants like amitriptylene or nortriptyline may be used to treat the overly excited nerves and give you some relief. You may be reluctant to take a medication that is an antidepressant, but remember that it is not being prescribed to treat depression. Antidepressants may cause other problems with your sexual response, so discuss any changes with your doctor.

Vulvar Vestibulitis

Vulvar vestibulitis is a chronic type of vulvodynia that may last for years if untreated. When you have vulvar vestibulitis, the *vestibule*—the area between your clitoris and perineum, including the area surrounding the opening to your vagina—becomes tender and red. The pain is usually described as stinging, burning, or raw and is usually localized in one or more distinct spots near the opening of your vagina. It may be difficult to touch or massage this area, and attempting to enter your vagina with a tampon, finger, penis, or sex toy may be impossible.

We don't know exactly what causes vulvar vestibulitis. Your doctor can sometimes make the diagnosis by using a cotton swab to look for areas that are abnormally sensitive to touch. If you imagine that the opening of your vagina is a clock face, it is most common to find tenderness at the five o'clock and seven o'clock positions.

There is no one treatment for vestibulitis that works for everyone, and a third of women will have spontaneous remission without treatment. You may find that some treatments work for you and not others. Sometimes combining two or more of the following treatments will do the trick.

> To prevent allergic reactions, stop the use of all soaps, deodorants, and perfumes on your vulva. Neutrogena or Basis cleansing

bars may be used for bathing, but make sure you rinse thoroughly. During your period, use only 100-percent nonchlorine bleached cotton tampons and pads, which can be purchased from the Internet site www.natural-woman.com.

For temporary relief of discomfort—long enough to allow you to have intercourse—soak a cotton ball in a local anesthetic (lidocaine) and place it against the tender area for 15–20 minutes before sex. This will make the area less sensitive to touch and may even make you feel numb; you should try to avoid contact between the lidocaine and your clitoris. By using a local anesthetic, you may find that you can safely have intercourse without pain, and since the inside of your vagina is not affected, you can enjoy stimulation of your G-spot, cervix, and other erogenous zones. You also may find stimulation of your clitoris to be pleasurable, though some women find that their clitoris also feels numb after using the local anesthetics. Be sure to use lots of lubricants for manual stimulation or intercourse to decrease friction. Apply an ice pack to your vulva to decrease any burning after intercourse.

Take calcium citrate supplements and decrease foods high in oxalate, an irritant excreted in your urine that can cause burning in some women. High-oxalate foods include nuts, wheat products, chocolate, citrus fruits, tomatoes, soy sauce, and spices such as ginger, pepper, and cinnamon.

Steroid creams, applied to the vulva, may help to reduce inflammation.

Biofeedback strengthens the pelvic floor and reduces pain of the vulva in some women.

Tricyclic antidepressants may alleviate pain by blocking some of the pain fibers that are in the vulvar tissue. These drugs may depress your sex drive, however, so the lowest effective dose should be used.

⚖ Doctors specializing in pain disorders may be able to inject a local anesthetic similar to lidocaine into the area for prolonged relief of pain.

⚖ Surgery to remove the tender tissue may be used as a last resort in women with severe pain that has not responded to any other treatments.

⚖ Though there have been no controlled studies, I have found acupuncture to be effective in some women with vulvodynia and vulvar vestibulitis.

⚖ Dealing with painful sex and the effect it may have on your relationship with your partner can be depressing, anxiety provoking, and distressing. You may feel hopeless as you try one treatment after another and fear that you will never be sexual again. Some women who have long-standing vestibulitis and painful sex also suffer from depression, in which case they should seek the help of a therapist.

Adhesions of the Clitoris

When secretions become trapped under the hood of your clitoris, the hood may stick to the clitoris and cause you pain when your clitoris becomes erect during arousal and during orgasm. Your clitoris may become so irritated that even touching it may be painful. Lichen sclerosus, a skin condition, also may cause your clitoris to become stuck to its hood.

Secretions can be washed away with a moist, cotton-tipped swab, and lichen sclerosus can be treated by medications prescribed by your doctor.

Pain During Penetration of the Vagina

Any of the conditions that cause pain when your vulva is stimulated can also cause pain when your vagina is entered by a finger, penis, or sex toy.

Vulvar vestibulitis in particular may cause severe pain and make sexual intercourse difficult or impossible.

Stiff Hymen

The *hymen* is a thin membrane that surrounds the entrance to your vagina. When you have intercourse for the first time, your hymen stretches or tears to accommodate your partner's penis. Some women have tight, stiff hymens that do not stretch and make any attempt to penetrate the vagina difficult and painful. You sometimes can soften the hymen by massaging daily with vitamin E oil. Occasionally, surgery may be needed to make penetration possible.

Vaginismus

Vaginismus is the involuntary spasm of the muscles surrounding the opening to your vagina. These spasms make entrance into your vagina difficult or almost impossible without significant force. Forced penetration may cause small tears around the opening of your vagina and lead to more spasms in response to the pain.

Vaginismus may be caused by fear of pregnancy, fear of pain, negative sex messages from childhood, a previous assault or rape, a problem in your relationship, or a painful first experience with sex. The problem may be present from the first time you have intercourse, or it may develop years later. Some women experience normal arousal and orgasm when they receive manual stimulation or have oral sex, but intercourse is painful and sometimes impossible. Vaginismus can make you feel depressed, frustrated, and inadequate.

To combat this problem, spend some time becoming familiar with your sexual anatomy. To learn to control your vaginal muscles, perform Kegel exercises daily and concentrate on contracting and relaxing your pelvic floor muscles. Your doctor may give you a set of dilators to help you learn to feel comfortable when something is placed in your vagina. When you have mastered the largest dilator, you may decide to include your partner in this process, allowing him to insert the dilator. When you're ready, you can move on to intercourse if you wish. The woman-on-top position will leave you in control of the depth of penetration and variation of movements.

If you do not wish to use dilators, you can use your fingers. Start with one lubricated finger and gradually advance to three. When you feel comfortable you can ask your partner to insert his fingers before advancing to intercourse.

A therapist is an essential part of the treatment of vaginismus and will help you to resolve the pain more quickly.

Vaginal Dryness

One of the first signs of arousal is lubrication of your vagina. Your vagina becomes wet to make it easier for a penis or finger to move inside. Sometimes, however, your vagina does not produce the moisture that you need for comfortable sex. Even massaging your vulva with a finger can be uncomfortable without lubrication.

There are many reasons why your vagina may be dry. Here are some common causes of vaginal dryness.

- If you are not adequately aroused, your vagina will remain dry. Women often need more time and more foreplay to become adequately aroused. Don't allow yourself to be rushed into intercourse before you are ready.

- Birth control pills and other medications may cause dryness.

- If you are postmenopausal and not taking estrogen, you may experience dryness. Some women notice decreased vaginal moisture beginning in their late thirties due to hormonal changes that occur as you enter the years leading to menopause.

- If you have a vaginal infection, your vagina will be swollen, irritated, and unable to lubricate well.

- If you are postpartum or breast feeding, hormonal changes may cause dryness of your vagina.

- Any medical problem that interferes with blood flow to your genitals may prevent adequate lubrication of your vagina.

A variety of sensuous lubricants are available to make sex more comfortable. Experiment and find the one that brings you the most pleasure. If you are menopausal, estrogen therapy or natural herbs will help increase vaginal moisture.

Lichen Sclerosus

Lichen sclerosus is a skin disease that causes itching and burning of the vulva. The vulva is easily irritated, and you may get tears and fissures when the skin is rubbed. Manual stimulation, oral sex, and intercourse may be painful. If left untreated, your labia minora may form adhesions or stick to your labia majora and clitoris. The opening to your vagina may become smaller.

Lichen sclerosus is treated with steroid creams (or ointments if the creams cause stinging). Some doctors also add estrogen or testosterone creams.

Scars from Episiotomy or Vaginal Tears

Scars from an episiotomy or vaginal tears obtained during childbirth can cause pain during penetration. It takes several weeks for complete healing of an episiotomy, but for some women, the pain and tenderness continue long after the wound appears to be healed. Massaging the scar daily with vitamin E oil and estrogen cream may make the scar softer and less tender.

An episiotomy or vaginal tear may also injure vaginal nerves. The injured nerve may form an abnormal mass called a *neuroma*. The pain caused by a neuroma is described as burning, aching, tingling, stabbing, and sometimes like an "electric shock." Sexual intercourse may be very painful. Some women have found that injections with local anesthetics have given prolonged or permanent relief from this pain.

Bicycle or Horseback Riding

Your pelvic nerves may be injured from pressure on your pelvis during frequent bicycle or horseback riding. You may develop an aching, burning pain that gets worse when you have sex. Some women also develop areas of numbness that interfere with their enjoyment of sex. You may need to take a vacation from these activities to see if the symptoms resolve on their own; if not, you will need to see a neurologist or pain specialist.

Pain with Deep Penetration or Thrusting

Inadequate Arousal

When you become aroused, your vagina becomes wet, and longer and wider at the top to accommodate a penis. If you have intercourse before you are adequately aroused, the penis will thrust against your cervix, uterus, and ovaries, causing discomfort. The pain is usually sharp but may have a burning quality. Changing your position may help, but try to spend more time building up to intercourse.

Mittelschmerz Syndrome

Mittelschmerz is German for "middle pain" and is the name for the pain that sometimes occurs in the middle of your cycle at the time of ovulation. When you ovulate, an egg is released from a follicle in your ovary. Sometimes the fluid that is released with the egg irritates the lining of your pelvis, causing pain and tenderness that can last for up to three days. If you have deep penetration during this time, you may feel a sharp, stabbing pain in your pelvis. Changing positions to decrease the depth of penetration may make you more comfortable; otherwise, you may have to skip intercourse altogether.

Endometriosis

You develop *endometriosis* when the tissue that is usually on the inside of your uterus finds its way to other parts of your body: most commonly your ovaries, the surface of your uterus, and inside your lower abdomen. When it is found within the muscle of the uterus, it is called *adenomyosis*. This tissue bleeds like the tissue that is found inside your uterus, causing pain during your periods. It also causes swelling and tenderness in your pelvis. Deep penetration may cause sharp as well as dull, burning pain that may increase when you have an orgasm and may linger well after sex is over.

Medications used to treat endometriosis include birth control pills and drugs that decrease your estrogen level. Sometimes surgery to burn or remove the endometriosis may be required.

Pelvic Inflammatory Disease (PID)

PID is an infection of your internal sex organs: your uterus, ovaries, and fallopian tubes. It is usually caused by sexually transmitted bacteria that make their way up from your vagina and cervix. When your pelvis is swollen and tender, deep penetration causes severe, sharp, stabbing, and burning pain that may linger for hours after sex is over.

Pelvic inflammatory disease must be treated with antibiotics. Your sexual partner must be evaluated and treated as well. It's wise to avoid intercourse until the infection has been adequately treated.

Ovarian Cysts

Cysts are fluid-filled sacs in your ovaries. Small cysts may not cause symptoms, but larger ones stretch the capsule that covers the ovary and may cause pain and tenderness. When you have deep penetration, the penis may thrust against the ovary and cause sharp, sometimes stabbing, pain. Some cysts spontaneously resolve; others must be treated with medication or surgery.

Pelvic Adhesions

Sometimes when you have surgery or a pelvic infection, you form adhesions where your pelvic organs stick to each other. When you have deep penetration during intercourse, your uterus and ovaries are jostled, and if adhesions are interfering with the free movement of your pelvic organs, you may feel pain. Try positions that limit the depth of penetration. If you continue to have pain, consult your doctor about the option of surgery to remove the adhesions.

Interstitial Cystitis

Interstitial cystitis is a chronic condition of the bladder that causes pain in the bladder and pelvis. You may feel the need to go urgently when your bladder feels full and you may urinate frequently—during the day and throughout the night. When a penis or finger presses against your inflamed bladder during sex, you may feel sharp, severe pain. For some women, the pain begins with arousal. It may be temporarily relieved by an orgasm but returns and may last for hours or days after sex is over. Changing positions so that the penis does not thrust against the bladder is helpful. In the woman-on-top and rear-entry positions, for example, the penis can be directed against the back wall of your vagina.

Doctors don't know what causes interstitial cystitis, but treatments include stretching the bladder with fluid, placing medications inside the bladder, or oral medications, including antihistamines, tricyclic antidepressants, and pentosan polysulfate sodium. Talk with your doctor about the best option for you.

If you are having pain with sex, don't be embarrassed to have a frank discussion with your doctor. There is no reason to suffer in silence. Most causes of painful intercourse can be successfully treated. A satisfying sex life is important to your quality of life—and you deserve it!

Chapter 22

The Vagina Dialogues: Frequently Asked Questions

Q. *Sometimes, after my husband and I make love, I notice some light vaginal bleeding. Is this normal? What can I do to prevent it?*

A. Bleeding after sex is a common complaint. And when it occurs, it can be frightening to you and your partner. *Any bleeding after sex should be evaluated by your doctor.* Though not the most common reason for bleeding after sex, cancer of the cervix, vagina, or uterus may present as postsex bleeding. Here are some of the common causes of bleeding:

Light bleeding: If you've had a wonderful experience, you're likely to be shocked to find a spot of blood on the sheet or pink secretions when you go to the bathroom. There are several possible causes for this kind of bleeding, the most common of which is vaginal dryness. When the vagina is dry, movement of the penis creates friction. As a result, your vagina becomes swollen, and tiny tears in the surface may produce a small amount of blood. Taking a warm bath and using lubricants next time may prevent this from reoccurring.

You may experience a similar occurrence if you are menopausal, have not had sex for a long time, or have very vigorous intercourse. It's also possible to get a vaginal injury from your partner's fingernails during manual sex.

If it is a day before or after your menstrual period, you may get a small amount of bleeding or spotting after sex. Movement of your uterus during intercourse or the contractions of your uterus during orgasm may cause loose blood and tissue in your uterus to be released.

If you have an infection of your vagina, you may have a small amount of bleeding. When the walls of the vagina are swollen, they are easily damaged during intercourse or manual sex play and may bleed.

Cervical problems, including infections and cervical *polyps* (small benign, grapelike overgrowths of tissue) as well as irritation from an IUD string, diaphragm, or cervical cap also may cause bleeding.

Heavy bleeding generally means there has been an injury to your vagina or cervix. Deep, vigorous thrusting during intercourse can tear the vagina, especially if you are menopausal or have vaginismus.

Again, any bleeding after sex must be evaluated by a doctor.

Q. *I often experience a burning sensation when I use the bathroom right after having sex. My friend says I might have a urinary tract infection. Is that likely?*

A. Burning with urination immediately after sex is a common complaint. Many women mistakenly assume they have a urinary tract infection. During intercourse, the urethra is massaged, compressed, and sometimes traumatized. As a result, it may swell and become sore. Vaginal dryness and vigorous prolonged intercourse or manual stimulation may increase the swelling and soreness, which may last for a couple of days. Using lubricants during sex can decrease trauma to the urethra. And soaking in a warm tub after sex may give you some relief.

Burning with urination that begins more than 24 hours after sex may be caused by a urinary tract infection or a vaginal infection. Sometimes it is difficult to determine the exact site of the infection, and it's possible to have infections of your bladder and vagina at the same time. In general, if the burning starts as soon as you begin to urinate and gets worse as your bladder empties, it is more likely to be a bladder infection. If the burning starts only after the urine touches your vulva, it is more likely to be an infection of your vagina or vulva. *See your doctor for an examination.*

Q. *I was recently diagnosed with a urinary tract infection, which I understand is somehow related to sex. Would you explain how such an infection could occur?*

A. *Urinary tract infections (UTIs)*—infections of the bladder and urethra—are common and often occur after sex. The *urethra,* the tube that goes from your bladder to the outside world, is short in women. When you have sex (intercourse, manual stimulation, or oral sex), bacteria that normally live on your vulva and anus are pushed into your urethra and then travel to your bladder. Symptoms of a bladder infection begin 24–48 hours after sex and include burning when you urinate, the need to urinate frequently, the feeling that you must urinate immediately or you will lose it, and sometimes blood in your urine. The burning usually begins immediately as you start to urinate and gets worse when your bladder is almost empty. *If you have signs of an infection, you should see your doctor.*

Using a diaphragm and/or spermicides increases your risk of a UTI. If you are using a diaphragm and having frequent urinary tract infections, you may need to change to another form of birth control. Your risk of an infection is higher after your very first act of sexual intercourse (the so-called *honeymoon cystitis*), the first intercourse after a long period of abstinence, frequent intercourse, and after prolonged and vigorous intercourse. Sexually transmitted infections can also cause urinary tract infections.

You can decrease your chances of getting a urinary tract infection by urinating before and soon after sex. Wash your vulva and the area surrounding your urethra before retiring for the night, and drink lots of water and unsweetened cranberry juice the day following a night of lovemaking. If you have frequent infections after sex, taking one antibiotic tablet immediately afterward may decrease your risk of a urinary tract infection. If you have intercourse again within the next six hours, there is no need to take another tablet. If more than six hours go by between episodes of intercourse, you may need to take another antibiotic tablet.

Q. *I often have trouble urinating right after sex. Should I be worried?*

A. When you become aroused, there is an increased flow of blood to your vagina, vulva, and clitoris. As a result, the area surrounding your urethra swells, making it more difficult for urine to flow from your bladder. Relax and give it time. Within a few minutes, the engorgement will shrink and urine will flow without difficulty.

Q. *Because of digestive problems, I am frequently constipated, which sometimes makes sex painful. What can I do?*

Sandra, age twenty-four, came to see me because she experienced bladder infections every time she had sex. She had been treated with multiple antibiotics without success. When questioned about sexual technique, Sandra said that her boyfriend enjoyed prolonged vigorous sucking of her clitoris, and despite some discomfort with this practice, she didn't complain. We reviewed female anatomy, and I used a mirror to show Sandra and her boyfriend, who had accompanied her for the visit, the close proximity of the urethra to the clitoris and explained what happens to the delicate tissues with vigorous sucking. I carefully recommended some changes in their technique of oral sex. Sandra called several weeks later to say she no longer experienced burning after sex.

A. Constipation can cause pelvic pain and discomfort during intercourse. The space between your rectum and your vagina is very thin. When you are constipated, hard stool can sit in your lower colon and press in toward your vagina. If you place your fingers in your vagina, you may feel a bulge on the back wall from hard stool. You may feel pain when you have intercourse, or you may feel pressure in your rectum. You may even feel as though you will have a bowel movement during intercourse, though this is unlikely to happen. Your partner also may complain that he "feels something" in your vagina during sex.

You can make sex more pleasurable by moving your bowels prior to sex, if possible. If not, choose positions where the depth of penetration is decreased. Meanwhile, treat constipation by increasing the fiber in your diet and drinking lots of fluid. *If these steps are not successful, see your doctor.*

Q. *Last week, in the middle of an amazing orgasm, I suddenly was gripped by pelvic cramping. Now I'm almost afraid to have an orgasm again because this pain was such a mood buster. What gives?*

A. When you have an orgasm, your uterus, lower vagina, and the sphincter of your rectum contract. The presence of some medical problems—such as endometriosis, adenomyosis, pelvic inflammatory disease, fibroid tumors, or ovarian cysts—can cause pelvic cramping during orgasm and interfere with your ability to enjoy sex.

The changes of menopause, including atrophy and shrinkage of your uterus, also may cause painful spasms of your uterus with orgasm. Estrogen replacement therapy may help but expect it to take several months of treatment before your discomfort improves.

Some women have cramping during and after orgasm while pregnant, especially in the last few months. *If the cramping lasts more than 30 minutes or is severe, call your doctor.*

Q. *Sometimes, the day after my man and I have had sex, I constantly feel wet. But I'm not turned on. What causes this excess discharge, and what can I do about it?*

A. If you have a high volume of secretions, you may notice a continuous leak the day after an evening of intercourse. Your own secretions increase during arousal and orgasm, and during ejaculation, a man releases about a teaspoonful of semen. The semen is thick at first but becomes thin and liquid while it's in your vagina. When you start to move around hours after sex, the combined semen and vaginal secretions begin to flow down your vaginal walls. But since your vagina is not a flat smooth surface, it may take a while for all of the secretions to move down the folds.

Wearing panty liners and changing them frequently the day after intercourse may make you feel more comfortable. Alternatively, you can place a tampon in your vagina after intercourse. Leave the tampon in for a couple of hours to soak up the secretions and semen and then remove it.

Q. *I sometimes get excruciating headaches right in the heat of passion. Could they be a signal of a serious health problem? What can I do to prevent them?*

A. Headaches are a well-used excuse for avoiding sex. We've all heard the complaint "Not tonight dear; I have a headache." But if you are one of the many women who suffer from headaches that come when you are in the throes of sexual ecstasy, this complaint is less than humorous. Sexual headaches may cause you to avoid sex altogether or hinder your ability to enjoy the experience. They usually aren't indicative of a serious problem, but you should see a physician, just to be safe.

There are two basic types of headaches that are brought on by sex. Both may be initiated by intercourse, masturbation, or oral sex. The first type of headache appears during sexual activity before orgasm. You may notice a dull, aching pain on both sides and in the back of your head. This headache is related to the so-called tension headache and may be brought on by the contracting and stiffening of the muscles of the face and neck during sex. As you become more sexually stimulated, the headache may increase in intensity. You also may notice tenderness in your scalp. These headaches may last only for a brief period or for several days. Taking ibuprofen (Aleve, Motrin) 1 hour prior to sex may be helpful. Biofeedback and muscle relaxation exercises or muscle-relaxing medications are sometimes necessary.

The second type of headache comes on just before or after orgasm. These headaches are severe, sharp, and throbbing, and may be located in the back, on one side, or on both sides of your head. Sometimes your whole head may throb. We don't know exactly what triggers these head-aches or why they occur during some episodes of sex and not others. It is possible that blood vessels in the head dilate, leading to this migrainelike headache. It is also possible that the increase in blood pressure that occurs with sexual excitement and orgasm contributes to these headaches in some women. You have a greater risk of developing this type of headache if you are prone to migraines in general. These headaches usually resolve within a couple of hours but may last much longer.

Your doctor may prescribe a migraine medication for you to take just before sex, or on a daily basis if the headaches are frequent. Alcohol con-sumption and recreational drugs may exacerbate these "orgasm head-aches." *If you have nausea, vomiting, weakness, drowsiness, stiff neck, double or blurred vision, or fainting—or if the headache lasts more than a few hours or is very severe—contact your doctor.*

Q. *Lately, I've been experiencing an annoying itch in my vaginal area immediately after sex. I don't think I have a yeast infection. What could this be?*

A. The most common cause of itching that begins just after sexual activ-ity is an allergic reaction. Contraceptive creams, foams, and gels containing nonoxynol-9 are the leading culprits. Condoms, particularly those made of latex, also may cause allergic reactions. Lubricants that are colored, flavored, and fragrant contain chemicals that your vulva may find irritating. You might cure the problem by using nonlatex condoms, avoiding spermicides that contain nonoxynol-9, and changing your lubricant.

Using a perfumed cream or spray on your vulva can cause problems when the perfume is pushed into your vagina during manual sex play or in-tercourse. Ask your partner about after-shave lotions and colognes that might have come into contact with your vagina and vulva during oral sex.

A rare cause of itching is an allergy to the proteins in your partner's se-men. If this is the case, using a condom should take care of the problem.

To calm the itching, sit in a cool bath. Applying a small amount of a mild anti-itch cream to your vulva might give you additional relief. *If the itching is severe, begins to spread to other parts of your body, or if you feel short of breath, call your doctor.*

NOTE: If itching begins two or more days after sex and is persistent, you may have an infection with yeast, trichomonas, or bacterial vaginosis (BV). See your doctor for evaluation and treatment.

Q. *I am fifty-two years old and—surprise!—noticing something new in my sex life. Unfortunately, it's not a pleasant surprise. Sometimes, I seem to be leaking urine during sex, which can be pretty embarrassing. Is this related to menopause? What can I do about it?*

A. Fear of urine leakage during sex can interfere with your ability to relax and enjoy the experience. Your instincts are correct: Incontinence of urine is more common during menopause as well as after childbirth.

You can decrease your chance of urine loss by urinating before sex and limiting fluid intake two to three hours before an intimate encounter. It's also helpful to avoid smoking and alcohol as well as caffeine-containing liquids such as coffee and tea, which act as diuretics and increase your need to urinate. Kegel exercises and other exercises for strengthening the pelvic floor may be helpful; sometimes surgery is necessary to treat incontinence.

Another cause of leaking urine is an overactive bladder. Your doctor may recommend a medication to relax your bladder and decrease the chances that you will leak. For menopausal women, estrogen therapy may be helpful. *See your doctor to make sure your incontinence is not caused by a bladder infection or other medical problem.*

Finally, if you lose urine only during sex and not at other times, you may be experiencing what is called *female ejaculation*. Some women secrete a liquid from their urethras during sex, often at the time of orgasm. Other women simply produce large amounts of vaginal secretions that make them and their partners feel wet. To make things more comfortable, place a few towels under you and try to relax. Remember that sex is a "messy business" where you share many fluids, including sweat, saliva, semen, vaginal secretions, and sometimes tears of joy. There is no reason to be embarrassed about a little additional warm clean fluid between loving partners.

Q. *The other night, I caught a cramp in my leg just as I was approaching the height of pleasure. Needless to say, the charley horse cramped my style. What could have caused that? How can I make sure it doesn't happen again?*

A. Getting a charley horse while in the throes of passion can bring a quick end to a pleasurable experience. Leg cramps are painful contractions of the calf or other muscles of the leg. They occur most commonly at night and last for seconds to minutes; some women find they get more leg cramps in certain positions. These kinds of cramps are more common in mature women and during pregnancy. The exact cause of leg cramps is unknown. Some medications, such as those used to lower cholesterol, may increase leg cramps.

You can prevent leg cramps by taking a warm bath and stretching before bed. Dehydration exacerbates leg cramps, so make sure you drink plenty of water every day. During a leg cramp, point your toes up toward your head, straighten your leg, and massage the muscle until it relaxes. *If you have frequent leg cramps, see your doctor for blood tests to check your electrolytes.*

Q. *Sometimes after my man and I have sex, I notice a distinct odor. It's not really unpleasant, just strong. What can I do to tone it down?*

A. Semen has its own distinctive odor, and when semen mixes with your vaginal secretions, a new odor is created. The odor is usually not foul or unpleasant. You may notice that the odor is different with different men, and with the same man at different times. Simple washing is usually all that is necessary. If you like, you can insert a tampon and leave it for a couple of hours to soak up the semen and reduce the amount of discharge and odor that you have following intercourse.

If you notice a foul odor after sex, check to be sure that you do not have a tampon or loose condom in your vagina (foreign bodies left in the vagina will cause a bacterial infection that causes a foul odor). *You should see your doctor to rule out a vaginal infection.*

Q. *I occasionally feel pain in my clitoris when I'm sexually aroused. Why is that?*

A. Adhesions sometimes occur when secretions are caught between the clitoris and the hood. During arousal, when your clitoris becomes engorged with blood and increases in size, these adhesions interfere with the enlargement of your clitoris and cause pain. If this happens, you can remove the secretions under the hood of your clitoris by using a moist, cotton-tipped swab. Gently pull back the hood and use the swab to wipe away secretions. You may find it helpful to sit in a warm tub of water as you remove the secretions. Sometimes massaging the hood also helps to loosen the secretions and makes them easier to remove.

Pain in the clitoris with arousal is sometimes caused by lichen sclerosus, a skin condition that causes the tissue of the vulva to become thin. Adhesions of the labia are common. When they involve the clitoris and labia, the clitoris can be almost buried by the adhesions. During arousal the clitoris enlarges, gets trapped, and causes pain. Lichen sclerosus can be treated with steroid creams. Estrogen or testosterone creams may be added to speed healing.

Q. *Sometimes, my PMS is so bad, sex is the last thing on my mind. How can I keep it from wreaking havoc on my sex life?*

A. Most women will have some of the symptoms of PMS *(premenstrual syndrome)* during their reproductive years. For some women, the bloating, breast tenderness, irritability, water retention, weight gain, mood swings, headaches, depression, and fatigue that come with PMS make it difficult to even think about sex. PMS can last from a couple of days to a couple of weeks. If depression, anxiety, and other mood changes are severe, you may have a more severe form of PMS called *premenstrual dysphoric disorder (PMDD)*.

Women with PMS (and PMDD) have been found to have less desire for sex, less frequent sex, and problems with orgasm during the days to weeks before their periods. If you are one of the women who suffers for half of each month, that doesn't leave a lot of time for satisfying intimacy.

There are many potential treatments for premenstrual syndrome. Your doctor can help you find the treatment that works best for you. I recommend frequent, small, and healthy meals, multivitamin/multimineral supplements, and calcium supplements. You should avoid alcohol, cigarettes, sugar, salt, caffeine-containing drinks, and chocolate during the two weeks before your period starts. Exercising at least five times a week increases your endorphins and makes you feel better. And make sure you get enough sleep. Acupuncture, yoga, and massage therapy are also helpful.

Some women find that taking low-dose (20-mcg) birth control pills alleviates many of the symptoms. Others have had success with natural progesterone creams or evening primrose oil.

The newest medical treatment is Sarafem (fluoxetine), an antidepressant (selective serotonin reuptake inhibitor) that is effective in many women with PMS and PMDD. Sarafem contains the same chemical as Prozac and may have the unwanted side effect of depressed libido and orgasm difficulty. Taking it only during the two weeks before your period—or taking a low dose—may prevent the sexual side effects.

Selected Resources

Ackerman, Diane. *A Natural History of the Senses* (New York: Random House, 1991).

Amias, A. G. "Sexual Life After Gynaecological Operations," *British Medical Journal* 2(1975): 608–9.

Anllo, Lisa. "Sexual Life After Breast Cancer," *Journal of Sex and Marital Therapy* 26(2000): 241–48.

Barbach, Lonnie. *For Yourself: The Fulfillment of Female Sexuality* (New York: Doubleday, 1975).

Baskin, Laurence, and Dale McClure. "The Fractured Penis," *Medical Aspects of Human Sexuality* (March 1990): 32–33.

Basson, Rosemary, et al. "Report of the International Consensus Development Conference on Female Sexual Dysfunction: Definitions and Classifications," *The Journal of Urology* 163(2000): 888–93.

Bullard, David, and Susan Knight. *Sexuality and Physical Disability: Personal Perspectives* (St. Louis: C. V. Mosby, 1981).

Cado, S., and H. Litenberg. "Guilt reactions to sexual fantasies during intercourse," *Archives of Sexual Behavior* (Feb. 1990): 49–63.

Castleman, Michael. "Recipes for Lust," *Psychology Today,* July/August 1997, pp. 50–56.

Chalker, Rebecca. *The Clitoral Truth* (New York: Seven Stories Press, 2000).

Chang, Jolan. *The Tao of Love and Sex* (New York: Penguin Books, 1977).

Crenshaw, Theresa. *The Alchemy of Love and Lust* (New York: Putnam, 1996).

Crenshaw, Theresa, and James Goldberg. *Sexual Pharmacology* (New York: Norton, 1996).

Daniluk, Judith. *Women's Sexuality Across the Life Span* (New York: Guilford Press, 1998).

Darling, Carol, and Kenneth Davidson. "Female Ejaculation: Perceived Origins, the Grafenberg Spot/Area, and Sexual Responsiveness," *Archives of Sexual Behavior* 19(1990): 29–47.

Davidson, Kenneth, and Linda Hoffman. "Sexual Fantasies and Sexual Satisfaction: An Empirical Analysis of Erotic Thought," *The Journal of Sex Research* (May 1986): 184–204.

Debusk, Robert. "Evaluating the Cardiovascular Tolerance for Sex," *American Journal of Cardiology* 86(2000): 51F–56F.

DeBusk, Robert, et al. "Management of Sexual Dysfunction in Patients with Cardiovascular Disease: Recommendations of the Princeton Panel," *American Journal of Cardiology* 86(2000): 175–81.

Dodson, Betty. *Sex for One: The Joy of Selfloving* (New York: Three Rivers Press, 1996).

Eichel, Edward, Joanne DeSimone Eichel, and Sheldon Kule. "The Technique of Coital Alignment and Its Relation to Female Orgasmic Response and Simultaneous Orgasm," *Journal of Sex and Marital Therapy* 14(Summer 1988): 129–41.

Engel, Beverly. *Raising Your Sexual Self-Esteem: How to Feel Better About Your Sexuality and Yourself* (New York: Ballantine, 1995).

Federation of Feminist Women's Health Center. *A New View of a Woman's Body* (New York: Feminist Health Press, 1991).

Fisher, C., et al. "Patterns of Female Sexual Arousal During Sleep and Waking: Vaginal Thermo-Conductive Studies," *Archives of Sexual Behavior* 12(1983): 97–121.

Friday, Nancy. *My Secret Garden: Women's Sexual Fantasies* (New York: Trident Press, 1973).

Gordon, Sol, and Judith Gordon. *Raising a Child Responsibly in a Sexually Permissive World* (Holbrook, Mass.: Adams Media, 2000).

Hatcher, Robert, James Trussell, Felicia Stewart, Willard Cates, Gary Stewart, Felicia Guest, and Deborah Kowal. *Contraceptive Technology* (New York: Ardent Media, 1998).

Heiman, Julia, and Joseph Lopiccolo. *Becoming Orgasmic* (New York: Simon & Schuster, 1988).

Hite, Shere. *The Hite Report: A Nationwide Study of Female Sexuality* (New York: Macmillan, 1976).

Inkeles, Gordon. *The New Sensual Massage* (Bayside, California: Arcata Arts, 1992).

Joannides, Paul. *Guide to Getting It On* (West Hollywood, CA: The Goofy Foot Press, 1999).

King, Bruce. *Human Sexuality Today* (Englewood, NJ: Prentice-Hall, 1999).

Laumann, Edward, John Gagnon, Robert Michael, and Stuart Michaels. *The Social Organization of Sexuality: Sexual Practices in the United States* (Chicago: University of Chicago Press, 1994).

Leiblum, Sandra, and Raymond Rosen. *Principles and Practice of Sex Therapy* (New York: Guilford Press, 2000).

Leitenberg, Harold, and Kris Henning. "Sexual Fantasy," *Psychological Bulletin* 117(1995): 469–96.

Lemack, Gary, and Phillippe Zimmern. "Sexual Function After Vaginal Surgery for Stress Incontinence," *Urology* 56(2000): 223–27.

Lobo, Rogerio. *Treatment of the Postmenopausal Woman* (Philadelphia: Lippincott, Williams and Wilkins, 1999).

Maines, Rachel. *The Technology of Orgasm* (Baltimore: The Johns Hopkins University Press, 1999).

Margolese, Howard, and Pierre Assalian. "Sexual Side Effects of Antidepressants: A Review," *Journal of Sex and Marital Therapy* 22(Fall 1990): 209–22.

Masters, William, and Virginia Johnson. *Human Sexual Response* (Boston: Little, Brown, 1996).

Masters, William, Virginia Johnson, and Robert Kolodny. *Heterosexuality* (New York: Gramercy Books, 1998).

Medical Letter. "Drugs That Cause Sexual Dysfunction: An Update," August 7, 1992.

Morin, Jack. *Anal Pleasure and Health* (San Francisco: Down There Press, 1998).

Mumford, Susan. *Healing Massage* (New York: Plume, 1998).

Nickell, Nancy. *Nature's Aphrodisiacs* (Freedom, CA: The Crossing Press, 1999).

Nunns, David. "Vulval Pain Syndromes," *British Journal of Obstetrics and Gynecology* 107(Oct. 2000): 1185–93.

O'Connell, Helen, et al. "Anatomical Relationship Between Urethra and Clitoris," *The Journal of Urology* 159(June 1998): 1892–97.

Panati, Charles. *Sexy Origins and Intimate Things* (New York: Penguin Books, 1998).

Papadopoulos, Chris. "Sex and the Cardiac Patient," *Medical Aspects of Human Sexuality* 64(Aug. 1991): 18–21.

Phillips, Nancy. "Female Sexual Dysfunction: Evaluation and Treatment," *American Family Physician* 62(July 2000): 127–36.

Rako, Susan. *The Hormone of Desire* (New York: Crown, 1999).

Rhodes, Julia, Kristen Kjerulff, Patricia Langenberg, and Gay Guzinski. "Hysterectomy and Sexual Functioning," *Journal of the American Medical Association* 282(1999): 1934–41.

Rose, F., and R. G. Petty. "Sexual Headache," *British Journal of Sexual Medicine* 24(Feb. 1982): 20–21.

Sardowski, Carol. *Sexuality Concerns When Illness or Disability Strikes* (Charles C. Thomas, 1994).

Sarrel, Philip. "Sexuality and Menopause," *Obstetrics and Gynecology* 75(April 1990): 26S–35S.

Seagraves, Robert. "Antidepressant-Induced Sexual Dysfunction," *Journal of Clinical Psychiatry* (suppl. 4) 59(1998): 48–53.

Sevely, Josephine Lowndes. *Eve's Secret: A New Theory of Female Sexuality* (New York: Random House, 1987).

Sexuality Information and Education Council of the United States. "Now What Do I Do?: How to Give Your Pre-teens Your Messages" (Washington, DC: GPO, 1996).

Sipski, Marcia, and Craig Alexander. *Sexual Function in People with Disability Chronic Illness* (Gaithersburg, Md.: Aspen Publishers, 1997).

Stanway, Andrew. *The Joy of Sexual Fantasy* (New York: Carroll and Graf, 1991).

Striar, Shama, and Barbara Bartlik. "Stimulation of the Libido: The Use of Erotica in Sex Therapy," *Psychiatric Annals* 29(Jan. 1999): 60–62.

Stubbs, Kenneth. *Erotic Massage: The Tantric Touch of Love* (New York: Putnam, 1998).

Warnock, Julia. "Female Hypoactive Sexual Disorder: Case Studies of Physiologic Androgen Replacement," *Journal of Sex and Marital Therapy* 25(1999): 175–82.

Whipple, Beverly, and Barry Komisaruk. "Sexuality and Women with Complete Spinal Cord Injury," *Spinal Cord* 35(1997): 136–38.

Winks, Cathy, and Anne Semans. *The New Good Vibrations Guide to Sex* (San Francisco: Cleis Press, 1997).

Zaviacic, Milan, and Beverly Whipple. "Update on the Female Prostate and the Phenomenon of Female Ejaculation," *The Journal of Sex Research* 30(May 1993): 148–51.

More Recommended Reading

Woman-Loving-Woman Sex

Loulan, JoAnn. *Lesbian Sex* (Denver: Spinsters Ink, 1988).

Newman, Felice. *The Whole Lesbian Sex Book* (San Francisco: Cleis Press, 1999).

Talking to Your Daughter About Sex

Haffner, Debra. *Beyond the Big Talk : Every Parent's Guide to Raising Sexually Healthy Teens—from Middle School to College* (New York: New Market Press, 2001).

Haffner, Debra. *From Diapers to Dating: A Parent's Guide to Raising Sexually Healthy Children* (New York: New Market Press, 2000).

Madaras, Lynda. *The What's Happening to My Body? Book for Girls* (New York: New Market Press, 1988).

Madaras, Lynda, and Area Madaras. *My Body, My Self for Girls* (New York: New Market Press, 1993).

Roffman, Deborah. *Sex and Sensibility: The Thinking Parent's Guide to Talking Sense About Sex* (New York: Perseus, 2001).

Internet Sites

For 100-percent organic cotton tampons and pads:

www.natural-woman.com

For sex toys, pelvic exercisers, and erotica:

www.babeland.com (Toys in Babeland: 1-800-658-9119)

www.goodvibes.com (Good Vibrations: 1-800-289-8423)

www.evesgarden.com (Eve's Garden: 1-800-848-3837)

www.grandopening.com (Grand Opening: 1-877-731-2626)

www.royalle.com (Candida Royalle's Femme: 1-800-456-LOVE)

Index

About the Author

Hilda Hutcherson, M.D., is the codirector of The New York Center for Women's Sexual Health at Columbia Presbyterian Medical Center and an Assistant Professor of Obstetrics and Gynecology at Columbia University's College of Physicians and Surgeons. A graduate of Stanford University and Harvard Medical School, she has practiced gynecology for more than twenty years. She is a frequent contributor to magazines, newspapers, and television. She is married and the mother of four.

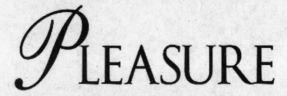
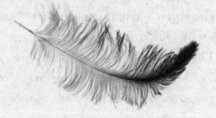